SOLVING (the) PALEO
E>Q=U+A:T×I-O<N

Dr. Garrett Smith
& Matt Stone

Victory Belt Publishing Inc.
Las Vegas

First Published in 2013 by Victory Belt Publishing Inc.

ISBN 13: 978-1-936608-27-0

Printed in The United States
RRD 0113

TABLE OF CONTENTS

INTRODUCTION

Matt Stone

It was a cold, dark, dreary, foggy night in South Florida when my phone buzzed. A rugged voice crackled in my ear. It was Dr. Garrett Smith. No, actually Garrett's voice didn't crackle at all and the weather was great. Florida for the win! I just thought all books were supposed to start out that way.

Garrett did call me (on an equally dreary and frigid night in Tucson, Arizona, I'm sure) and said that he wanted to put together a book sharing the insights the two of us accumulated while working in the health, nutrition, and fitness fields. Garrett's experience comes from his naturopathic medicine practice and days as a competitive power lifter; my experience stems from seven years of independent health research and extensive communication with the large online following I built up during that time.

After chatting for a while and really thinking about the kind of book we wanted to write, as well as what our expertise and personal health histories had led us to believe, we mutually decided that the book's main purpose was to "keep people from f%#@ing themselves up."

This book is not directed at those who sit around guzzling Mountain Dew by the keg or who hit McDonald's on their way to work every day. There are plenty of books written for them. The reader we're interested in targeting is the health fanatic in pursuit of six-pack abs and a clean-as-a-whistle diet—the ones with the best of intentions and the worst results.

In today's Internet age, with thousands of studies coming out every nanosecond, gurus everywhere promising perfect health and ways to "disease-proof" yourself by following a few simple eating rules, and fads and trends coming in and out of vogue all the time, the casualties of modern health fanaticism are shockingly abundant. From the eighteen-year-old in the Netherlands who took his testosterone levels to near zero trying to obtain the perfect physique to my childhood buddy tearing his quadriceps muscle in an unfit CrossFit workout, I've seen the biggest losers in the perfect health game. Garrett has seen his fair share as well.

So this book is a far cry from a motivational piece trying to inspire you to cut every last evil, gluten-filled noodle out of your diet. This is not a book full of tips for squelching your cravings for all of those pesky favorite foods of yours. This is something else entirely. This is a real-life guide to being as healthy as you can reasonably expect to be in our modern world in a way that is balanced, safe, and practical.

Why the title *Solving the Paleo Equation*?

There are many reasons we chose this title. For starters, there is a raging fever circulating in the world today over the Paleo diet—the idea that if we modern humans do our best to eat only the types of foods available to our ancestors tens of thousands of years ago, we too will have the supposed great health that these early hominids experienced. However, in real-world practice, this approach is extremely limited, and in order to make this "equation" work, many more of the fundamentals of good health need to be added.

Second, Paleo is like any diet craze, in that the more people who are invested in one narrow approach, and the more they are sold on the premise or ideology of that craze—whether it's scientifically valid or not—the greater the fallout. By *fallout* I mean the damage that's done when people fail miserably despite firm adherence to the rules and discipline. That damage includes tons of health problems, from digestive issues to hormonal problems to loss of energy, sex drive, mood stability, and other things that make the difference between a good and a bad daily life experience.

Stated more bluntly, we see the Paleo diet as it is commonly practiced, as well as some of the exercise recommendations that typically accompany it, as one of the most common causes of health problems in health-conscious people today. Garrett and I have seen it again and again. And we have experienced it for ourselves, which is what enabled us to see outside that box and take our understanding and expertise much further.

We don't adhere to any philosophy or trend. Garrett is on the Garrett Smith diet. I'm on the Matt Stone diet. Garrett goes to the gym for his GarrettFit workouts. I practice MattFit. Ultimately, all our experience, both personal and professional, has led us directly toward understanding and emphasizing proper function—function over philosophy. And when it comes to improving function, individuality throws all rigid rules, and even "scientific breakthroughs," completely out the window.

Thus, the book you are about to read is all about balance, self-driven customization, and monitoring basic biofeedback for signs of improved function. If that concept sounds simple, then good—it is! Hopefully, like us, you will find the simplicity refreshing. We won't be supplying you with rigid and harsh rules, lists of good and bad foods, or impossible exercise routines. No need to retreat to a cave in the hills. We are minimalists; small changes translate into big results. We are all about the fundamentals: stress management, moderate exercise (outdoors when possible), deeper and more restful sleep, and a metabolism-supporting diet. Those few things will deliver 90 percent of the benefits to any health-conscious person.

Our hope is that once you've finished this book you will understand how your body works and end your addiction to finding the perfect diet and health plan—that nonexistent panacea that will solve all your health problems once and for all. You don't need the Internet to tell you how to be healthy; the answers are inside you. Once you know how to listen to the cues of your body, you won't need an outside authority to tell you how to live and eat.

This is yet another reason why we chose to write this book with the ancestral health theme of the Paleo movement—our evolutionary heritage is in us. Your body is the best doctor, the best nutritionist, and the best personal trainer you could ever hope for. Our bodies regulate energy intake and output. They regulate thirst and fluid balances. They regulate our need for exercise as well as our need for rest and sleep. We have all the instincts programmed in us to manage our bodies well. Unfortunately, with so many ideas about how much exercise, food, and water we need, modern humans have gotten into the increasingly bad habit of intellectually interfering with our instinctual programming. We let books and blogs and magazine articles tell us how and when to eat and exercise, or how much water or rest we need. In other words, it's not about getting back in touch with your prehistoric diet, it's about getting back in touch with the prehistoric *you*.

Also, we hope you'll rediscover the true fundamentals of health, no longer confusing what are relative minutiae for matters of life-and-death importance while completely ignoring the simple, timeless basics. There are a million different health tips, tactics, and tools floating around in the world today. You can't partake of them all without driving yourself crazy, and becoming flat broke and socially isolated in the process. Our goal is to identify what is of primary importance to your health—what you should give precedence to—and what is secondary and, therefore, relatively inconsequential.

We sincerely hope this book empowers you as no other health book ever has, delivering great results without telling you to go against yourself in any way. That's our intention, and that's what we believe to be the future of how human beings honor and care for themselves.

Enjoy!

PART

1

[S-T>R+E·S=S]

Matt Stone

Chapter 1
DEFINING STRESS

Stress is not a specific reaction.
The stress response is, by definition, not
specific, since it can be produced
by virtually any agent.

—Hans Selye, *The Stress of Life*

Stress! Eek! Deadlines, babies crying in the night, rush-hour traffic, the death of a loved one, divorce, bills, debts, arguments . . .

Those are the things most people think of when they hear the word *stress*. They are, to be sure, some major stressors. But the subject of this section is certainly not stress in this classical and narrow sense. When we say *stress,* we mean "stressors," and when we say *stressors,* we mean anything that ignites the stress circuitry of the body.

Is stress inherently bad? No. It's necessary. Without stress we don't grow, we don't develop, and we ultimately don't fulfill our highest physical, mental, and emotional potential as human beings.

Is stress inherently good? No. It's harmful, destructive, and ultimately delivers the final blow to our bodies and minds that ushers us toward the big red EXIT sign in the sky.

That's right. Stress is neither good nor bad. It is what it is: Stress giveth, stress taketh away. It's important not to think in black and white terms when it comes to the human body, as you will repeatedly hear in one form or another throughout this book. There are no heroes and villains. Everything depends on the circumstances, the dose, the duration, and other factors.

Rather, what we want to do is steer you toward the idea of balancing your life appropriately and being cognizant of the total stress burden you are under, as well as understanding the recovery side of the equation. It must be balanced for best results.

One of the most overused but simplest and most powerful examples of this concept is that of exposing your skin to the sun's ultraviolet rays. Each of us has our own natural threshold for sunlight. There is tremendous variance from one individual to the next. There is also a large variance in sun tolerance, depending on the time of year and how much sun you've been getting lately. Thus, even in one individual the tolerance for sunlight is always changing.

Let's say Billy Vanillaskin has a tolerance for direct sunlight of fifteen minutes. Each minute of sun exposure is sun stress. Billy can handle up to fifteen minutes of this stress without inflicting so much stress as to cause sunburn. If he goes out for fifteen minutes his skin responds by getting a little darker and becoming more resilient—expanding his sun tolerance by several more minutes. He can keep doing this, always staying within this threshold, until he has a nice tan and can stay out in harsh sunlight in the middle of the day for a couple of hours.

This is a perfect example of stressing the body, prompting the body to adapt to that stress and get stronger and more resilient over time. Without that stress, Billy's skin would have continued to be pasty and hypersensitive. In this case, stress works as a positive, beneficial stimulus.

However, if Billy goes out on his first day for two hours without undergoing this adaptation process, uh-oh. That could mean second-degree burns and major skin damage. His skin might even become *more* sensitive to sunlight for a long, long time after so sudden an onslaught. This is an example of too much stress and a great deal of damage being done—it's not positive or beneficial at all.

Simple enough, right? But it's an important foundation for the ideas about stress we are working with. You want stress, but it has to be *manageable* stress that's within your personal threshold; otherwise, you risk serious damage. Additionally, the type, strength, and duration of stress that it takes to cause destruction, rather than regeneration, is highly variable from one individual to another. And that's not all. How you perceive a stressor can make a fundamental difference, too. For example, if you are running while playing and having fun, the stress you experience (*eustress*—literally, "good stress") is totally different from that experienced by the self-loathing dieter who is grudgingly facing unwanted exercise on a treadmill just to burn off some calories (*distress*). As phrased by Hungarian physiologist Hans Selye, the godfather of understanding stress on the physiological level:

> During both eustress and distress the body undergoes virtually the same negative stimuli acting upon it. However, the fact that eustress causes much less damage than distress graphically demonstrates that it is "how you take it" that determines, ultimately, whether one can adapt successfully to change.

Let's leave stress's effects behind and start looking specifically at stressors. This should help you think beyond the simple definition of stress that you've got currently floating around in your head. Becoming aware of all forms of stress is the starting point for making any kind of personal stress assessment at any given time or at any stage of life.

Chapter 2

TYPES OF STRESSORS

As Selye claims, stress can be produced by virtually any agent. So the following list is by no means exhaustive. No list could ever comprehensively encompass the myriad things that elicit a stress response. Below are some of the major ones, as well as the most common, especially among the health-conscious. We'll call these the Dirty Dozen (and hopefully that won't cause any cliché stress).

1. Psychological stress This is obviously the biggest and the baddest of the stressors; it also comes in the greatest variety. Psychological stress is particularly powerful because our psyche has a very strong impact on our physiology. It can also stick around, sometimes for years, and become chronic and debilitating, unlike the acute yet relatively insignificant stress of, say, some granny driving like Stevie Wonder, her car swerving in slow motion toward your Mini Cooper (the most common source of acute stress in the state of Florida). A painful event from even decades ago can still affect your body, especially if you frequently revisit the experience in your mind. Psychological stress comes in the form of holding grudges, anxiety, divorce, being overly stressed about work, relationship dissatisfaction, doing a job you hate, financial stress, babies crying in the night, dealing with the tragic loss of life of those close to you, social anxiety, body image insecurity—the list goes on and on. If a memory or thought can trigger a strong emotion any time you think about it, it's probably a great source of stress.

2. Diet stress Most of you probably wouldn't consider dieting as a source of stress, yet for some it's the mother of all stressors. Chronic

calorie deprivation and carbohydrate restriction are the most extreme dietary stressors, and they are stressors that no amount of meditation or spiritual awakening can overcome. There are other diet stressors, like restricting a food that you wish you could eat—denying your cravings can be a huge stress. Likewise, continually gorging on a food that you don't tolerate well can create an inflammatory reaction and is also a source of dietary stress. Binge eating in response to your self-imposed dietary restrictions is another stress, often topped with guilt that lasts well beyond the physical distress. Eating, in general, is one of the primary de-stressing activities, so you have to account for not only causing stress but also missing out on one of your primary stress relievers.

3. Inflammation stress There is a massive amount of research on the huge role that inflammation plays in most diseases. Well, guess what? Stress heightens inflammation and inflammation heightens stress. And there is no doubt that anything that sets off inflammation will also initiate a release of inflammatory mediators like cortisol, which is the body's main stress hormone. Ever take hydrocortisone or prednisone for a nasty allergic reaction? These are pharmaceutical variations of our own cortisol and provide an anti-inflammatory effect. But keep in mind that chronic inflammation can lead to chronic hypercortisolism—too much cortisol. Chronic infections, of which there are endless varieties (including the many familiar viral and bacterial infections as well as common things like gum disease or dental infection), can trigger this high inflammation, chronic high-stress situation. There is also very strong evidence that modern human cells are primed for producing overzealous immune and inflammatory responses in general—hence the epidemics of food allergies, asthma, autoimmune disease, and other hyperinflammatory conditions. Much more on this to come in Part Two: Nutrition because much of this type of inflammation can be improved with simple dietary changes.

4. Sleep stress Some research suggests that the average night's sleep a century ago was around nine hours. Today we average

closer to seven hours, and many people get far less. Chronic sleep deprivation is certainly known to be a major source of chronic stress, and, like harsh dietary restriction, this is particularly detrimental because not only are you causing stress by missing out on sleep, you are missing out on a primary antistress tool. It's a double whammy. (Yes, I just said *double whammy*. I try to say it any chance I get.)

5. Medication stress There are many medications that can cause chronic stress on several fronts, due to their active ingredients and their actions. Even some antidepressants (Prozac and friends) are known to raise cortisol levels. There are also many habit-forming substances, such as alcohol and nicotine, that may lower cortisol in the short term but over time lead to a higher overall stress burden. Prescription, over-the-counter, and recreational stimulants—from Adderall to Sudafed to weight loss pills to your morning coffee—are being used in greater and greater amounts worldwide. Stimulants are yet another way of digging your spurs into your stress system.

6. Exercise stress Exercise is a form of stress. There's no question about that. In the right amounts and in the right context (when you are eating lots of food, carbs in particular; you're getting good sleep; and you have low to moderate stress levels), exercise is one of the highly beneficial stresses. But, as Garrett will get into in greater detail, there is no question that exercise can also turn sour. And that's because fewer and fewer people in this day and age (and fewer still among those with a health and fitness fetish) are exercising in the right quantity, dosage, and context. While exercise has undeniably wonderful attributes in a general sense, for many individuals it is one of the greatest, if not *the* greatest, sources of stress.

7. Light stress There's no doubt that one of the most "un-Paleo" things we do in the modern world is totally mess around with normal and natural light exposure. Bright light raises cortisol. This may sound like a bad thing, but a peak in cortisol in the morning hours when the sun is bright and shining is normal and healthy.

In the modern world, however, we have managed to extend the number of hours we're exposed to bright light with our shiny new gadgets. We now keep ourselves awake, bright lights a-blazin' and cortisol a-soarin', in a "wired" state after dark. I'm talking primarily about those glowing, luminous boxes like computer screens and televisions. At best, we miss out on much-needed sleep and have trouble naturally winding down—which is stressful. At worst, this late-night light can increase total stress hormone exposure. There's no doubt that higher cortisol levels in general increase the risk for developing many health problems, such as the constellation of factors that comprise metabolic syndrome (insulin resistance, high blood pressure, high blood glucose, abdominal fat storage, etc.). There is also evidence that constantly being bathed in electromagnetic frequencies (EMF) from all the electrical gadgets and appliances that surround us takes a toll, increasing stress. While it is definitely *not* our intention to make you paranoid enough to retreat into the wilderness stark-naked and barefoot to avoid the ravages of modernity, going to bed closer to sunset, sleeping in as dark a room as possible, and, at the very least, dimming your computer monitor after dark are all fairly practical interventions that are powerful stress reducers.

3. **Seasonal stress** Winter in and of itself is a stressor, and the human body simply doesn't function at its peak mentally, emotionally, or physically during cold, dark winters. While I don't necessarily encourage you to move to the tropics to avoid this, it's certainly good to become aware of seasonal stress and adjust your diet, exercise, and lifestyle patterns accordingly. It may be customary in January to starve oneself and jump on a big, unsustainable exercise kick to burn off holiday excesses, but it is definitely an example of poor timing.

4. **Sexual stress** While this could be filed under the broader category of psychological stress, there are some physical considerations to take into account as well. Not getting enough sex is very stressful, but so is getting too much. In a world full of constant sexual bombardment through television, advertisements, and, of

course, pornography, many people—men especially—put themselves under great stress by engaging in excessive sex and masturbation. This may sound ridiculous, but sex uses a lot of reserve energy, and it can get drained, just like anything else. In addition, too much stress crushes sex drive and function.

10. Irregularity stress One thing overlooked in today's chaotic world is the importance of regular rhythms and patterns. There is even some evidence that having a consistent meal schedule rather than an erratic one promotes a healthy metabolic rate, cholesterol levels, and more. In real-world practice, the simple act of having a regular and consistent schedule for exercise, meals, bedtime, and waking time can be very helpful in stress management. As Scott Abel, one of the fitness industry's leading experts, says, "The body thrives on regularity." Anytime there is chaos instead of consistency, our bodies are much quicker to dive into a stressful alarm state.

11. Noise stress Loud and obnoxious noise is another often-overlooked stressor. If it has the power to annoy, you can be sure it's a trigger of the stress response. Construction workers who fail to use ear protection at noisy job sites experience dramatic rises in cortisol. While you may have little control over your exposure to noise in your own life, it is still a potent source of stress for some. The good news is that most can become desensitized to noise over time and have a minimal physical reaction to it.

12. Stress-list stress Reading long lists of things that can trigger stress triggers stress. Before, you were unaware of how harmful stress is and the many ways it is entering your life. Now, you are deathly afraid of developing "the Beetus" and having your leg amputated a couple decades from now because you own a television, winter is approaching, and you have a toothache. You are staying up even later now researching diabetes prevention on the Internet and scouring late-night infomercials for magic cures. While this rant is obviously going above and beyond the call of duty to lighten things up a little bit, it is a good lesson to learn in general. Don't read too much about all the harmful things in our world, in our

diets, and in everything that is more or less normal these days. Being weird and isolated from everyone in a state of health paranoia is a huge stress, too. You might consider backing off your fierce health and nutrition research habit. Ignorance is sometimes bliss in this regard. If you are going to read health stuff, dim the screen on your e-book reader or laptop when you do it. You know, light stress and all. And as Kent was instructed by God in the movie *Real Genius,* "Stop playing with yourself!"

Now you can identify a few of the more prevalent kinds of stress. In the next chapter we'll get into something even more useful: how to assess your overall stress burden through common indicators.

Chapter 3
STRESS INDICATORS

As a reminder, we want the beneficial, strengthening effects of stress. A challenging mental task can make us smarter; a tough experience can mature us emotionally; a challenging workout can make our bones and muscles stronger and make our lungs and hearts function better. But how do you know when you are getting figuratively "sunburned" by all the stress in your life—maybe even buckling under the weight of it? Your body is a good messenger of this. Here are ten of the most common signs that your body and mind are under too much stress and that you have exceeded your stress threshold.

1. Insomnia When the stress system becomes hyperactive, adrenal hormones start to surge in unusually high amounts at night. This can mean difficulty falling asleep, or it can mean waking up between two and four in the morning feeling overly alert or anxious (maybe you're sweating or your heart is racing or palpitating) and having difficulty falling back to sleep.

2. Fatigue Stress is very energizing; it makes us feel alert, just like a cup of strong coffee. But too much stress on a chronic basis is very depleting and wears you down, leaving you feeling wiped out, especially during the first half of the day.

3. Drowsiness after meals Insulin is released in response to food and shuts down adrenal activity. If you are "strung out" on stress hormones and eat a big meal, you may get extremely drowsy or have a crash type of feeling after eating—especially after big, heavy meals that combine lots of fat, protein, and carbohydrates.

Generally, the higher the stress hormone levels before the meal, the bigger the post-meal crash.

4. Low sex drive Sex drive and function peak in times of plenty. Under stress, the energy allocated to reproduction typically falls precipitously.

5. Frequent urination Stress hormones are diuretic, meaning they make you empty your bladder often. If you urinate frequently during the day or at night (*nocturia*) and have to urinate several times in response to even small amounts of water, or if you feel strong, sudden urges to urinate at various points during the day, your stress system may be overactive. If you are inducing frequent urination by intentionally guzzling down excessive quantities of water, this too is very stressful, as you will soon discover.

6. Excessive thirst or dry mouth Coupled with frequent urination—and exacerbating it—are the dry mouth and excessive thirst that often accompany chronic hypersecretion of stress hormones. If you are urinating frequently with very clear urine and your thirst is still not satisfied—it might even seem to get worse the more you drink—you are likely in a chronically overstressed state.

7. Anxiety or depression If you are experiencing either of these—and likely it's both, since the body oscillates between these two mental states under chronic stress—it's a sure sign that your stress levels are at debilitating highs.

8. Exercise intolerance If strenuous or even moderate exercise makes you ill and completely wiped out for days, your stress levels are either too high or you're doing more exercise than your body can withstand at this time.

9. Cold hands and feet When stress hormone levels are elevated, the blood vessels in the extremities (hands, feet, ears, tip of your nose) close up and restrict blood flow, resulting in cold hands and feet at various points during the day, or chronically if you are particularly stressed.

10. Menstrual irregularity The menstrual cycle is usually affected by stress, which causes progesterone levels to fall and negatively affects period flow—it gets too heavy or too light, or stops altogether if stress is severe. Also, when progesterone is lacking toward the end of the menstrual cycle, symptoms such as cramping and PMS may intensify. Stress may also disrupt the normal rhythms between the luteal and follicular phases of the menstrual cycle, leading to increased testosterone and the masculinization often seen with the disorder known as polycystic ovary syndrome (PCOS).

This is a short list of the ways in which excess stress manifests itself. There are many other ways, including the development of allergies and intolerances; autoimmunity; frequent colds, flu, and other infections; dry skin (particularly around the hands, feet, and scalp); tooth decay or bone loss; infertility; hair loss; and many others. There are some weird ones, too, like lactating when you're not pregnant. Digestion is also usually pretty terrible, since it is not a prioritized function during stress. In fact, it shuts down and can lead to constipation, delayed stomach emptying, bloating, and more, as we will discuss in Part Two: Nutrition.

It can get worse, too. The adrenal glands have a breaking point, which can lead to adrenal fatigue and the inability to produce enough adrenal hormones (much worse than too much, especially considering that DHEA, a hormone with countless beneficial effects, is produced by the adrenal glands) or Addison's disease, which is the true flatlining of the adrenal hormones. In the latter case, even dressing yourself or brushing your teeth feels like getting jousted by a gladiator.

By now you should be feeling a little more knowledgeable and empowered when it comes to stress. You know some of its primary triggers as well as some of the ways that being overly stressed surface in the body and mind. If everything you've read in this section sounds unfamiliar, consider yourself lucky. But remember what you've read as you may encounter some of these problems in the future and need to know how to interpret them. Even aging itself causes stress; as we get older, stress hormones increase in proportion to antistress hormones like DHEA, testosterone, progesterone, and T3 (thyroid hormone). Few escape the stress monster completely for a lifetime and, more importantly, as you go through the many stages of life, you have to continually adjust your health "equation" to meet your varying needs and thresholds.

While the rest of the book is dedicated primarily to antistress activities, the next chapter outlines a few helpful ways to combat stress in your life.

Chapter 4
DE-STRESSING TOOLS

Exercise, diet, and sleep are the ultimate weapons of stress reduction, and we'll get into those in greater detail later in the book. In the meantime, here are some very simple yet effective ways to combat stress in your daily life.

1. Neutralize your negative emotions Easier said than done, right? It's an ongoing practice, but any work you do toward achieving greater emotional neutrality regarding past and present events and circumstances can be quite liberating. I view emotions as feelings that arise whenever we view something as being more positive than negative or more negative than positive. There is, of course, an entire movement dedicated to the power of positive thinking. You shouldn't delude yourself into thinking that something "bad" is "good," but you can use your conscious mind to change your perspective on things tremendously.

   An exercise I highly recommend is sitting down with a piece of paper and writing out a list of the biggest negative emotional triggers that you have accumulated in life thus far. They could stem from a negative event, a person in your life you perceive as negative, or a perception you have about yourself and your shortcomings. To help lessen the chronic stress-triggering effect of the accumulated baggage of certain experiences or people you have dealt with, next write out all the positive ways in which your life has changed because of that person or event.

   What most people find, if they dig deep enough, is that a painful experience or situation has actually paid big dividends in other areas, steering their lives in ways that they wouldn't change for the world. Being sick as a child was something I always resented, but now I can see that this difficult experience is one of my primary motivations for becoming a health researcher and writer and dedicating my life to better understanding how the body works. In turn, I've helped others to climb out of similar situations. It couldn't have happened any other way. I had to experience poor health to later be motivated to learn as much as I could about human health. When I realized this, I went from resenting this life experience to being very grateful for it. This is just one simple example.

In essence, what you are doing in this exercise is going beyond the simple pain and suffering you might have experienced and the limited view you had of it to acknowledging the full spectrum of how that experience shaped your life, for better and for worse. If you never think about them, you'll forever experience pain, suffering, and ultimately stress from experiences originally perceived as negative. Yet often it is the greatest tragedies that lead us to find our purpose in life and fulfill our highest potential. So try spending some time neutralizing past and present traumatic events to the extent that you feel the emotions revolving around them lessen. Ultimately, the goal is to feel pretty grateful for the life you have, and have had, and for how it has made you who you are today.

At first, you will feel that there is no positive side to a horrible event or evil person. That's an indicator that your emotions surrounding it are highly charged and in need of resolution. But keep looking until you find one. It is always there. Your mind will resist this process with absolute ferocity, but press on. As you neutralize the negative feelings surrounding an event or person, you can begin to see how it made you who you are.

To do this exercise more thoroughly I highly recommend reading Dr. John Demartini's *Quantum Collapse Process* or working with a specialist who can guide you through dissolving emotional baggage in this manner, such as Bella Dodds, one of the site authors at www.180degreehealth.com.

2. *Slow your brain-wave activity* The frequency of your brain waves directly stimulates the nervous system. In a world where people zone out on four hours of television daily, I hate to discourage active brain use. But for those with overly active brains that are continuously humming along and generating high-frequency beta waves all day and night, activities that encourage a more relaxed alpha-wave state may be quite therapeutic. There are many ways to produce more alpha waves and fewer beta waves. Meditation is probably the most common therapeutic tool for this. Light yoga or something similar can work, too. Generally, anything that allows you to feel relaxed, including snuggling up to a movie in the evening as opposed to thinking obsessively about all the tasks awaiting you at work, could be just the right thing to help you unwind. This can help you naturally wind down for sleep as well, that wonderfully de-stressing activity of which modern humans are so starved.

I know of what I speak. I do most of my writing (definitely a beta-wave activity, since it requires great focus) late at night and have difficulty calming down my mind and going to sleep. In my case, it's worth it because the quality of my writing at night is astounding. It's as if I have managed to wring the sweet nectar of Shakespeare's *Hamlet* into mesmerizingly informative prose on this very page, which could possibly explain why you are weeping harder and harder with tears of inspiration the deeper you travel into this book. My unprecedented writing skill aside, here are a few more ways to calm those beta waves.

3. *Take a vacation* Not everyone can afford a trip to some exotic location, but by *vacation* I don't only mean getting on a cruise ship or boarding a plane—though I'm not discouraging those options. Any effort to create downtime, even if it's just taking a week off from work and riding your bike every day, is worthwhile.

Even better than a vacation is actively redesigning your life in a way that makes it more sustainable or enjoyable or inspiring. Easier said than done, but there's no stress greater than living a life that doesn't inspire you or doing unfulfilling work day after day after day. While it may seem like pie in the sky from your vantage point, if you were to truly start spending more time doing what you really want to do with your life, you would quickly find that things come together much more easily than when you try to force yourself to do what "makes sense" for your career path or whatever you find yourself stuck doing. There's never been a better time in history to forge your own career path doing exactly what you find most interesting.

Hell, there's a young kid on YouTube who makes thousands of dollars a month filming videos with Barbie dolls. I'm in communication with dozens of Internet entrepreneurs who are making anywhere from a few thousand to a few hundred thousand dollars a month, and I would bet that their skills and abilities are no greater than yours. The only thing that separates them from the rest of us is their strong desire to escape the rat race and follow their dreams and interests. If you take even half the time you spend daydreaming about doing something else with your life and put that time toward actually following through on it, you'd probably be well on your way within a year. Even if you didn't, your life would still be a lot better with a creative side hobby displacing your feelings of trapped helplessness.

I could go on about this for hours, because I'm one of those people who followed through on something to the point of not having to "work" anymore. I will spare you that sermon, but know that doing what you love for a living is a lot easier than doing what you hate. You will simply go much further, much faster, and amass more valuable skills, knowledge, and expertise, when applying all your efforts toward the things you naturally have an affinity for doing.

4. Spend more time outdoors The indoor environment is a stifling and emotionally oppressive place. Spending time outdoors, on the other hand, puts most people into a totally different, and much more calm and serene, state of mind. Physically, spending time indoors—a place filled with all kinds of electronic gadgets, appliances, and more—appears to subject the body to a variety of

stressful electromagnetic frequencies (EMFs). Garrett will discuss this in more detail in Part Four: Sleep and Recovery, but being outdoors and in contact with the earth is inherently de-stressing for many reasons. While it's often a hard thing to do, I have never once regretted dragging myself outdoors. It is always uplifting and calming to the senses. In a world of exotic cures and elaborate theories, simple things like walking in a park or on a beach are often forgotten. Maybe advice to get outdoors isn't flashy or complex enough to dazzle anyone—it's certainly not very marketable. But it should be emphasized, not overlooked, in any conversation on health and psychological well-being.

5. Get warm Many things in the body are two-way operational. By that I mean that if A causes B, then B can often cause A as well. You will recall that earlier I mentioned that having cold hands and feet is a prominent sign of having an overactive stress system. You can stop this stress in its tracks by simply warming up the body, which naturally shuts down the stress system. Think hot baths, saunas, down comforters, and sunbathing. You have certainly felt how calm and relaxed you are after getting really warm in a hot bath or Jacuzzi. It's worth seriously considering making a hot bath a regular part of your regimen, especially if your feet are very cold when you go to bed.

6. Laugh Laughter is a great de-stressor. You're welcome. (That's me acknowledging your gratitude for the boundless hilarity I possess, which is so delicately and artfully woven into the pages of this book. I happily share it with you.) What's the use in being the funniest person ever to live if I can't share it? The only time laughing has backfired and increased stress levels for me was recently when I stayed up until four a.m. watching clips from the show *Just for Laughs,* a Canadian gag show (damn that light stress and sleep loss!). Canadians know a thing or two about the de-stressing effect of laughter. They wouldn't survive in that miserable, godforsaken wasteland of a country without a good sense of humor. If that show is still not enough to make you laugh (unlikely) and my

writing has ceased to entertain you (really unlikely), Dave Chappelle doing stand-up comedy is one thing that never gets old.

Well, that's it. Those are the only conceivable ways to lower your stress levels.

No, of course not. Lowering your stress levels can happen in an infinite number of ways. Odds are, if something makes you feel calm and at ease, whatever that may be for you personally, it can be used as a de-stressing tool. Much more to come later in the book as we discuss the most powerful of all de-stressing tools: sleep and antistress nutrition.

Chapter 5

THE METABOLISM-STRESS CONNECTION

Okay, enough lists, for crying out loud. I hate lists as it is, and so far this book is one list right after another. Before we move on, the last thing that is of great importance for you to grasp is the close connection between stress and metabolism.

In the past, I have compared the relationship between stress and metabolism to a tug-of-war. What sends metabolism up sends stress down. What sends stress up sends metabolism down. While a stress biochemical like adrenaline will indeed increase the rate of metabolism—the entire basis for why "thermogenic fat burners," or weight loss pills, contain massive doses of stimulants—this increase in metabolism is fleeting and isn't stimulated by the same mechanism that usually governs metabolism, the thyroid gland. In fact, there is evidence that under conditions of stress, the thyroid gland slows down and even atrophies. In experiments carried out by Robert McCarrison, enlargement of the adrenal glands (a sign of hyperactivity) was always accompanied by atrophy of the thyroid gland. The same thing is observed under starvation conditions, and even just a regular restriction of calories in the form of a diet increases cortisol and decreases T3, the primary metabolism-driving hormone.

Thus, stress is not necessarily just stress. There appears to be some metabolic control of the secretion of stress hormones. If you are doing something that reduces your metabolic rate, you can expect much higher levels of stress hormones to be circulating in your bloodstream. Likewise, if you raise your metabolic rate, this can be a massive de-stressor. We'll discuss this at great length in Part Two: Nutrition because achieving a tangible increase in metabolic rate with dietary manipulation has long been the primary focus of my research.

Another interesting connection that is worth mentioning here is that the symptoms of low metabolism are the same as the symptoms of the condition known in alternative health as "adrenal fatigue." Of course, adrenal fatigue manifests as a decrease in adrenal hormone activity, but this often occurs after long-term abuse and a chronic elevation of adrenal hormones. Still, the symptoms of the two are virtually indistinguishable. Look at the following graphic from the book *Taking Up Space* by Amber "Go Kaleo" Rogers.

Physical Symptoms of Adrenal Fatigue	Physical Symptoms of Anorexia/Starvation
+ fatigue	+ fatigue
+ insomnia, sleep disturbances	+ insomnia, sleep disturbances
+ poor digestion	+ poor digestion, constipation
+ poor immunity, frequent colds, flu, infections	+ poor immunity, frequent colds, flu, infections
+ low blood pressure	+ low blood pressure
+ sensitivity to cold	+ sensitivity to cold
+ poor recovery from exercise	+ muscle weakness, poor recovery exercise
+ anxiety, depression	+ anxiety, depression
+ irritability	+ irritability
+ poor memory, brain fog	+ poor memory, brain fog
+ loss of appetite or excessive appetite, cravings	+ loss of appetite, cravings, fixation on food
+ reproductive hormone dysfunction	+ amenorrhea, reproductive dysfunction

Before diagnosing yourself with Adrenal Fatigue, be sure that you are not, in fact starving yourself. gokaleo.com

From my observations, the scenario is pretty straightforward. Stress lowers metabolism, and as metabolism gets progressively lower, stress hormones get progressively higher. We're not talking small increases: Peaks in adrenaline can be thirty to forty times higher when metabolism is being suppressed through overzealous exercise, dieting, work stress, sleep loss, and other primary stressors. After prolonged hyperelevation of stress hormones, the adrenal glands become congested and inflamed (seen in autopsy in virtually all of both McCarrison's and Selye's experiments), and they start to fail to produce adequate amounts of the adaptive stress hormones. An overabundance of stress hormones is bad. Not enough is *much* worse! With true adrenal fatigue—also known as Addison's disease—the symptoms are extremely debilitating.

Anyway, that's enough bad news about stress. Do what you can with some of the de-stressing tools mentioned earlier. They will likely have a bigger impact than you think.

PART

2

[NUTRITION]

Matt Stone

Chapter 6
FUNCTION FIRST

Maintaining health is a fragile and dynamic process. What a person needs at any given moment to stay balanced and well functioning is highly variable. I shouldn't even need to point out the obvious limitations of what's commonly considered the "Paleo diet"—including the many subcategories of the Paleo diet like low-carb or raw Paleo—or of any diet for that matter. It is indeed a step back in time to adhere to a firm dietary prescription of any kind and hope to meet the dynamic and variable needs of the human body on any given day, at any stage of life, or under any circumstance.

When you think about the broader needs of an organism and its cells, it becomes clear that a change in diet is extremely powerful. But it also should be clear that there can be an infinite number of recipes to return a person to proper function. In my many years of exhaustive communication with other diet researchers, I have found that while diets can indeed cure diseases, the diet that makes one person well can make another person sick. Along the same lines, a diet that yielded a miraculous health turnaround for someone can later make that same person sick again.

People have different needs at different times. A diet that can bring someone back into balance can also overshoot that balance and create an imbalance. This is all complicated further by the fact that feeling great in the short term doesn't mean that you are improving your health. That massive euphoria you are feeling from a new diet or lifestyle change could be a surge in stress hormones that will ultimately lead to an epic crash a few months or years later.

In short, there is no dietary prescription for everyone—or even for one person. There is no magic diet, but a change in diet can still be quite magical.

Rather than theorize as to what the perfect diet is, as so many have foolishly done before me (and I have done before myself)—followed by laying out one of those mind-numbing diet plans for you to blindly follow with fingers crossed—I would rather use this section to get you thinking more about how your body works and less about the minutiae of nutrition.

I find it much more appropriate to present a set of physiological goals and let you use these goals to manipulate your diet, lifestyle, and other influences on your health in a way that maximizes your functioning and your overall health.

Basically, the sum of all your health practices (nutrition being one of the primary foundations of that, of course) should lead to proper function. The problem is defining *proper function*. Everyone has a yardstick for good health. Some see it in digestion; others in the skin and teeth or in a lean, muscular body. Most doctors consider complex blood tests to be the true marker of health. I have my own yardstick, and without getting into too much of a Nerdy McNerdfest, let me explain how I created it.

Throughout my investigations into nutrition and human health over the last decade or so, I have encountered one recurring theme again and again: metabolism. Metabolism is not necessarily how many calories you can eat without gaining weight, although in some individuals this can be a clue. Rather, when I say *metabolism,* I'm talking about metabolic rate. When I say *metabolic rate,* I mean the rate at which energy is produced at the cellular level. The metabolic rate cannot be measured solely by how many calories a person consumes because people come in a variety of shapes and sizes. A big person will almost always have a higher metabolic rate than a smaller person if you don't adjust for size. But when you do adjust for size, you find that smaller people generally have much higher metabolic rates than larger people; that is, they produce more energy per pound of lean body weight.

A clearer example might be to compare two dogs of different sizes. I recently saw a Giant Bull Mastiff that looked like a friggin' bear. I'll bet the owner has a second job just to pay to feed that thing! Yet a tiny Chihuahua, which might make a single Mastiff meal last for a whole week, probably has a much higher metabolic rate. The Chihuahua's respiratory rate is higher, its body temperature is likely higher, its resting pulse rate is much higher, it has much higher energy levels, and so on.

And, contrary to what many believe about metabolism and longevity, this higher metabolic rate results in fewer health problems and a significantly longer life span. In fact, if you compare two members of the same species (the only fair comparison), the smaller-sized member typically lives longer—that's right, the one with the higher, not the lower, metabolic rate.

Most health researchers adhere to the old theory that if you have a higher metabolic rate, you'll just burn up more quickly and die at a younger age. This is a popular and logical-sounding theory, but it's inaccurate. It's similar to those other scientific fables about carbohydrates causing diabetes and saturated fat causing heart disease. Um, no.

But this isn't a debate about longevity. Whether a high metabolism increases or decreases your rate of aging is of little consequence. What really matters is that you are physically and mentally performing at your peak for as many years as possible. None of us in our right mind should sacrifice decades of mood stability, high energy levels, great sex drive, good-quality sleep, and that kind of thing for a few extra years in our eighties or nineties.

So, with that behind us, why do I think metabolism is so important? Even going so far as to claim that it is the single most important metric to base one's dietary and lifestyle decisions upon? Well, I could try to whip up some studies and attempt to prove it to you that way, but unfortunately that wouldn't be any more convincing than some other book with a jillion studies supposedly backing up a different point of view.

Besides, few scientists understand the full spectrum of metabolism. Some track calorie consumption to make that assessment; others look at respiratory rate or thyroid hormone levels. There's not much congruence there, and only one metric in isolation doesn't show anything with much real-world value. I'd rather tell you exactly—albeit in a very abbreviated way—how I came to believe, through the convergence of many things that convinced me beyond any doubt, that metabolic rate is of great value in avoiding, and reversing, many common health problems, both minor and major. Metabolic rate is far from the only factor in good health, of course, but it should be considered the foundation on which health is built. Here's how I came to believe that.

I've always been fanatical about health and a bit of an overachiever in the physical realm. Early on, these tendencies expressed themselves as a constant struggle to eat less and exercise more. You know that one, right? It started innocently enough and quickly morphed into a great source of inner turmoil: me against my instincts and urges.

I won some battles, but many times I failed. My body's energy-regulating system turned out to be quite a formidable adversary. Unfortunately, with each failed attempt to eat less than I wanted to eat or to exercise more than I wanted to exercise, my stress level increased. With determination renewed and recharged, I would go at it again, hell-bent on even more severe self-punishment. In a story of revenge and redemption, I made myself out to be an underdog in an epic battle against that troublesome body of mine. I was tired of losing to those hunger pangs and that innate desire to just watch some television or listen to music or some other woefully unproductive pursuit.

The battle started in my early teens and kept going and going and going on a long, escalating journey involving things like—well, I won't give too much away just yet. And even though I noticed lots of new and wonderful health problems emerge during this time—like asthma, severe seasonal allergies, tooth sensitivity, and crippling back pain from a degenerating disc in my spine—nothing really got my attention until my sexual gland failed me for the first time. Previous aches and pains were, if anything, heightened motivation to transcend my earthly body's desires, just weakness leaving the body or whatever. But my schlawinkydink? This was serious!

Did I mention that this happened just after I turned twenty-one? Yes, ol' Humplestiltskin went soft in the throes of passion with a tender, voluptuous, giggly nineteen-year-old *Star Wars* fanatic, the perfect erectile stimulator for an American male born in the seventies. (I mean, there were little Yoda figurines all over her room! The lightsaber should have been fully brandished!) This inauspicious event occurred after one of my more self-punishing excursions, specifically, a three-day, 325-mile bike tour riding up one of the steepest roads in all of the Rocky Mountains (think 4,000-foot continuous ascent) pulling a kid cart with fifty pounds of supplies. To top this off, the temperatures were below freezing, with winds over 30 mph.

I figured this bike tour ordeal would be the final blow—the kill shot—in the war on myself. But in response to this grueling ordeal, I spent the next couple of weeks doing basically nothing and eating horrifying amounts of food. I vividly remember going to a Baskin-Robbins in Durango, eating a double scoop on a sugar cone, pausing briefly, then ordering another.

Being the wise individual I am, I realized that this was just what the body needs to rejuvenate itself in response to brutal physical tasks. I then went on to make peace with myself.

Not really. That would be the ending to a novel perhaps, but I, of course, responded to my ice cream binges by deciding that the only reasonable solution was to *never eat ice cream again*!

It was clear that ice cream was my weakness. Ice cream was the artillery used by the infidels. I had to cut off the supply completely if I wanted to win this war. And I did. I didn't touch so much as a spoonful of ice cream for a few years. Victory!

Shortly after—sing along with me if you know this one—I happened upon a powerful book talking about the evils of ice cream by none other than the son of Mr. Robbins of Baskin-Robbins himself. Ice cream killed his family! So he started a war against ice cream and everything else enjoyable to eat. This totally made sense to me at the time, and I went on to spend more than a half-decade as a vegetarian. Thank you, John Robbins. I'll always look back at those years—bent over in pain from the gastrointestinal distress of eating beans, lentils, and soy for nearly every meal—with great nostalgia.

And I haven't even gotten to the climax of this saga yet!

Yes, I kept going and going to greater extremes to "strike back" at my hunger and laziness with more outrageous feats of physical endurance and food deprivation. Turns out that a little lightsaber malfunction is just the least of the consequences of wrecking one's metabolism.

Operation Metabolism Destruction came to its inevitable conclusion with a fifty-day trip into Wyoming's fabled Wind River Range. I intentionally did not bring enough food and took no sugar at all, since that had always been my weakness. With these meager supplies, I planned on covering huge distances over tough terrain in harsh weather.

This is where my real education on human metabolism began. As my body fat disappeared my emotions became unstable, my bowels seized up, and my eliminations went from three large logs per day to just a few pebbles of black charcoal twice a week. I got unbearably cold, my hair started falling out, my sex drive completely vanished, and I spent all day and night daydreaming of food and writing out elaborate menus and sketching kitchen designs. I urinated incessantly—up to ten times per hour after my watery breakfast porridge—and laid awake at night, tossing, turning, and shivering until four a.m.

It was as powerful a lesson in human physiology as one could ask for in life. I learned about the consequences and symptoms of a low metabolism. I learned that eating less and exercising more didn't result in the happily-ever-after utopia I had envisioned.

Since I had broken myself, and the hunger in my belly was no longer a sign of "doing good" but cause for anxiety and horror, I had to find another way.

I did.

My relationship with my body rapidly changed from one of constant war to one of great alliance and trust. In fact, I started daydreaming about creating an educational foundation called the Body Trust. It was the germ of what later became a passionate personal research project.

I had much to learn, and learn I did. As I started relentlessly researching starvation, metabolism, hypothyroidism, and related topics, a much clearer picture started to form. More importantly, I began encountering more and more people with very familiar symptoms. I also learned about lots of new symptoms that I didn't experience. Mark Starr's book *Hypothyroidism Type 2* has a chapter called "Symptoms" that spans eighty-five pages! Lo and behold, it turns out that the generation of energy in each of our cells—the metabolic rate—influences every organ, every system, and every function in a pretty dramatic way.

Most importantly, as I began learning the ins and outs of controlling metabolic rate through diet and lifestyle interventions—something I later dubbed "Rest and Refeeding"—I got to see thousands of people put it to the test, raising their metabolism based on some of the simple indicators outlined later and overcoming low metabolism–related health conditions pretty consistently. My theories have been put to the test, and they have been confirmed by real, living, breathing people who overcame their low metabolism-related health conditions. These people integrated these changes—not in a lab, but in real life. All these things combined have convinced me that metabolic rate is a central player in a very large percentage of health conditions, minor and major.

Metabolism isn't everything. I've certainly progressed beyond the immature stage where cure-alls and Santa Claus exist. (The jury is still out on the chupacabra—mangy coyote my ass!) It is very important, though, and the type of people that Garrett and I were hoping to reach with this book, passionate health seekers exploring strange diets and superhuman exercise programs, are exactly the type most likely to be lowering their metabolic rate in an attempt to be healthy. Hey, if someone wants to smoke, drink alcohol, and eat at Mickey D's every day, that's fine. But seeing so many people put so much effort into bettering their health and having it all be in vain is what gets me upset.

Of course, many things besides your health and nutrition practices influence your metabolic rate. A lot of it is hereditary or due to other things that may have happened in your past. Maybe you got hit by some of those stressors we talked about or other factors. Regardless of what has converged to set your metabolic rate where it currently resides, I think it's about time to talk about metabolic rate, some prominent indicators of the overall quality of your metabolism, and some very important nutritional mistakes that you could be making right now that are working against you. By the time all is said and done, we will have laid out a few important nutritional foundations and guidelines for you to start incorporating into your life while tracking the results. But, before jumping in, let's take a quick look at the Paleo diet specifically, since I know that many of you reading this have been seduced by it.

Chapter 7
THE PALEO DIET

To be frank, to solve the Paleo equation, you must first subtract the Paleo diet. The Paleo diet, for those of you who have been hiding in caves and aren't familiar with it, is basically an attempt to eat the way our ancestors ate, within reason, before the dawn of agriculture. I would describe it in greater detail if I could, but nobody is really sure what the Paleo diet is, really, as there is a wide variance in macronutrient ratios and diet composition of various eaters calling themselves "Paleo" all over the world. For the most part, it is a diet free of grains, most dairy products, and as many über-modern, refined, and processed foods as possible.

Does the Paleo diet have some virtues or merit? Sure! I ask you to subtract it, and any diet ideology for that matter, from the equation because all diet ideologies are limiting. You cannot be rigid in your thinking if you hope to keep up with the changing, flowing nature of your body. Today's miracle diet won't necessarily work for you tomorrow. When you change, your diet must change to meet the demands of the new and different you, and that's often impossible when you are deeply entrenched in one narrow way of thinking.

I have written an entire book dispelling the "isms" of the Paleo diet. For the purposes of this book, I will give you just a few things to consider. This is not an attempt to debunk it, but more an attempt to just loosen up the rigidity of your thinking a bit, as I know there are some die-hard Paleo enthusiasts reading this book. Here are some of the basic tenets that are far from being definitively true.

[1]
We are genetically identical to our ancestors.

Not by a long shot. Most scientists believe that humans are currently undergoing the most rapid genetic changes that we, as a species, have ever experienced. And that's without even considering the biggest wild card of all: epigenetics, the study of gene expression or cellular phenotype. We have epigenetic buttons that are pushed in response to changes in previous generations, and that largely determines how genes are expressed. The human body has an elaborate mechanism for adapting to dietary and environmental changes. It leaves us with more questions than answers about what is the true "genetic blueprint" for any individual. That's why trying to mimic the diet of our ancestors or a traditional group of people like the Inuit or the Masai tribe in Kenya, for example, doesn't work in my experience. Genes forged tens of thousands of years ago have little to do with what our immediate needs are or what diet yields the best overall results.

[2]
Natural is always better.

The dogma for nutritionists and health nuts has become: "If it's *natural* it must be superior." But often it's the *unnatural* that gives a species a big leg up. Certain climates and regions are limiting. Resources are limited. Take the simple example of yeast. Yeast doesn't thrive in the real world to the same degree that it thrives in a laboratory. In a lab, you can create the ideal temperature, the perfect moisture level, and the ideal combination of fuels and nutrients, and a yeast population will proliferate as it never could in the harsh elements of the real world. Yeast multiplies so quickly that, under perfect conditions, it could blanket the world in a matter of weeks. Any species, humans included, could similarly thrive under ideal artificial conditions.

An even better example would be cooking. At some point, it was "natural" for humans to subsist on raw foods exclusively. But cooking breaks food down and allows us to both consume greater quantities of food and absorb a higher percentage of nutrients in that ingested food. Cooking food, an unnatural process, is what author and biological anthropologist Richard Wrangham believes is the most important advance in human history, allowing us to flourish and propagate our species in ways that were impossible when we only ate raw food. Basically, all creatures grow larger and multiply faster on cooked food, not because it's natural, but because it's better than natural, or *supranatural.*

Yet another example is the development of the rapidly absorbed and hyperrefined maltodextrin and dextrose, corn-based carbohydrates included in the sports drinks many athletes consume before, during, and/or after exercise. These are far from natural or "whole" foods, and yet when it comes to superior athletic performance, muscle growth, and faster recovery, they are far more effective than beans, fruit, and other slow-digesting carbohydrates.

There are plenty of other examples. Don't get me wrong: I'm not saying Cheetos are awesome because they are unnatural, but trying to mimic the harsh dietary and lifestyle conditions of our distant ancestors with blind faith that it is better because it is somehow more "natural" is definitely built on some false premises.

[3]
Carbs raise blood sugar and insulin levels, leading to insulin resistance, diabetes, and obesity.

The Paleo movement, thankfully, is slowly moving away from this viewpoint, which it clung to in the beginning. It is just outright false. Carbohydrate consumption does not cause a chronic rise in blood glucose or insulin, and insulin spikes do not cause the pancreas to fail or insulin resistance to develop. That's simply not the etiology of metabolic syndrome, which is still not fully understood and is hotly debated. Simple theories like this one may sound good and make sense to the uninformed public, but it was passed around like a rumor with little real validation of its truth. It would take a full dissertation to delve into the real etiology of insulin resistance, but this one you can file away with other bogus theories. In fact, carbohydrates may help protect against these disorders, and it makes a lot more sense from a metabolism point of view—and certainly from an exercise point of view—to run the body primarily on glucose.

[4]
We have not adapted to eating foods like grains and dairy products.

In fact, we *have* adapted, and the human body has undergone many adaptations that suggest this is so—like producing lactase into adulthood and producing very high amounts of salivary amylase for breaking down starchy foods. Not everyone fares well with a lot of grain and dairy, and people should be informed about the possibility of eating a diet where these foods are minimized to see if, indeed, they are causing problems. This rarely has anything to do with our evolutionary history, however; it has a lot more to do with a person's digestive health, hyperinflammatory immune system, and other individual flaws and weaknesses. Most people do great on such foods and find, just as our ancestors did, that there are many advantages to having a ready supply of carbohydrates and nutritious dairy products throughout the year. Dairy, especially, is a prime example of a supranatural substance in the human diet. Hey, if you don't tolerate it that's okay. But you need not look for some prehistoric explanation for why your nose gets stuffy when you eat too much cheese.

[5]
Modern Paleo is how our ancestors ate.

Attempting to eat like our ancestors is an attractive idea on the surface. However, under closer scrutiny, there are many fine details left out. Early humans inhabited nearly every region of the globe, each with its own unique flora and fauna. They ate what was available to them, which varied from region to region and from season to season. With so many unknown variables, simply picking up some coconut, sweet potatoes, walnuts, bananas, beef, and salmon at your local supermarket and pretending that this truly mimics an ancestral diet is ludicrous. Bananas are a modern hybridized fruit that is no more Paleo than French bread. The same can be said of just about all varieties of fruits and vegetables available in supermarkets. Paleo produce wasn't anything like the options available today. It was small, fibrous, and full of alkaloids and plant poisons, making them highly indigestible. Furthermore, salmon is a cold-water fish that lives at high latitudes while coconut is a warm-weather crop that thrives in the tropics. Our ancestors certainly *never* combined these two food items at a meal. Essentially, we can't re-create a truly Paleo diet in the modern world, and those who have convinced themselves that how they are eating is at all similar to the food environment fifty thousand years ago are deluding themselves.

Anyway, hopefully this demonstrates some of the flaws that fly in the face of the powerful logic that seems to underlie the Paleo diet. Embrace our modern food supply. Generally speaking, we can be healthy and vibrant eating modern fruits, vegetables, grains, and dairy products. Health doesn't require extremism or harsh dietary restrictions. In my experience, both the practice and the mind-set of eating a specialized diet with long lists of no-no foods is completely out of sync with the overall experience of health and vitality.

If you need to cut some foods out of your diet, that's fine. Nobody can eat everything; nobody likes everything. But dietary restrictions should be kept to a minimum and never used as a first line of defense. For some of us, there are digestive, metabolic, and inflammatory precursors that make many foods intolerable. Fixing those core problems will do much more to increase your vitality than just cutting foods out of your diet—that will get you a little relief but doesn't fix the root problem. I have helped many people overcome food allergies and intolerances, so I know it's possible and very liberating and empowering for those who succeed. Neurotic food avoidance rarely leads to radiant long-term health, except in very rare cases.

As a final word on the Paleo diet, one of the most important considerations when it comes to prehistoric humans, and all animals really, is that there was little, if any, intellectual interference between instinct and the food and fluids ingested. This is something that has been almost completely overlooked by Paleo supporters, as far as I know. I thought it worth bringing to your attention because it's not just *what* early humans ate as much as it is *how* they ate. When food was abundant, as it usually was, humans had the ability to select foods based on what they desired without the knowledge of dietary good and evil.

Studies on humans who are able to select what and how much they want to eat, without worrying about what they should or shouldn't be eating or drinking, show that we are remarkably adept at maintaining a healthy weight and much more. (Yes, there really are studies on this; most of them can be found under the Resources tab at www. intuitiveeating.com.)

In my experience working with thousands of people, I have come to one very powerful conclusion again and again: We shouldn't stifle our instincts and impulses with strict regimens and powerful ideologies. I'll get into this more later, but before there were diets and rules about eating, people ate what they craved. They didn't, for example, eat potatoes when they wanted steak, or eat steak when they wanted potatoes. They didn't eat less than they wanted to eat, nor did they eat more than they wanted to eat. They drank not because they were instructed to stay hydrated but because they were thirsty. They then stopped when their desire to drink went away. They didn't set alarm clocks or take stimulants when they were tired. They slept when it was dark and when they were tired—at least when times weren't stressful.

If there is anything that we still carry today that is an extremely powerful remnant of our evolutionary fine-tuning, it is this: We have all the tools to regulate energy balance, hydration levels, and macronutrient balance inside us. Try eating just a couple of apples for breakfast; you'll likely be gnawing your arm off by noon because all the nutrients we need are not found in two measly apples. Our bodies detect this and trigger us to fill in the missing gaps. These mechanisms are so fine-tuned that just a small bite of something salty increases thirst within seconds; our body is programmed to maintain the proper balance of sodium and water.

Today we have an abundance of ideas about what we should and shouldn't be doing with our food choices, and this, to me, is totally out of touch with our ancestral programming.

Overriding your natural cues, especially when it comes to thirst and hunger, is dangerous and carries with it a great deal of collateral damage. Paleo is in you! Your body knows exactly when it needs certain things, like water, salt, sugar, meat, fat, sleep, and sex. The sooner you stop trying to intellectually interfere with a system that already works, the sooner your health will start to improve. I'm excited to share more of this self-guided empowerment in the pages ahead, because the ultimate diet guru is in you. It's your little inner caveman/woman.

Now let's get back on track and dig deeply into this metabolism idea.

Chapter 8

METABOLISM: THE FOUNDATION

M etabolism, as I've mentioned, isn't the be-all and end-all. But it's the foundation on which health is built. Consider a few of the critical ways in which your metabolic rate influences the basic systems of your body.

Digestion

Metabolism is a primary controller of your bowel transit time, which is the amount of time it takes for the food you eat to come out the other end. A healthy transit time is about twenty-four hours. The mammal with the lowest metabolic rate is the tree sloth, with a body temperature of 91°F and a transit time of thirty days! Because your metabolism controls bowel transit time, constipation is one of the first things to be relieved when the metabolic rate goes up. More stool is passed, its moisture content is higher, it is easier to expel (no straining), and it typically has less odor because your poop hasn't spent as much time putrefying in the gut. Less time in the intestines also means less fermentation of fiber, sugars, and starches (so less gas, bloating, and flatulence), as well as less time for bacteria and other microbes to multiply and proliferate, particularly in the small intestine, which should be almost completely sterile. (According to Mark Pimentel, the head of gastroenterology at Cedars-Sinai Medical Center, bacterial overgrowth of the small intestine is thought to be the predominant cause of irritable bowel syndrome.) One by-product of bacteria, called *endotoxin,* notably triggers the cascade of events that leads to increased systemic inflammation.

DR. GARRETT SMITH & MATT STONE

Once bowel transit time is improved, many people experience improvements in the digestive disorders related to straining and constipation—like diverticulosis, hemorrhoids, and anal fissures.

But there's more: With a reduced metabolic rate, you are more likely to have a delay in stomach emptying. The most severe form of this is called *gastroparesis,* which leads to, among other things, a great deal of discomfort and bloating for hours after meals, as well as acid reflux and heartburn.

Once you begin to raise your metabolism, the body increases its production of a hormone called *gastrin,* which strengthens digestive secretions and fosters greater digestive prowess; *furnace* or *incinerator* are words often used to describe the way your stomach feels once these improvements set in.

The relationship between digestion and metabolism is a great example of how much of an influence metabolic rate can have on seemingly unrelated functions.

Energy Levels

The sloth is a wonderful segue for this topic, as this hypometabolic creature has extremely low energy levels, low muscle mass (the lowest in all the animal kingdom), sleeps up to sixteen hours a day, and is, well, a sloth! Raising your metabolic rate makes you less and less sloth-like over time. Your energy levels start to rise; your desire and threshold for physical activity rises; the quantity of sleep you need to feel rested decreases; drowsiness after meals disappears; and you experience an increase in overall vigor and vitality.

As we age, our mitochondria—the central producers of metabolic energy at the cellular level—accumulate a lot of damage. This slows the metabolic rate over time. This is the primary reason that our energy levels are on a downward trajectory as we get older. So anything we can do to delay or reverse this degradation is beneficial to the overall quality of our lives.

Sex Drive

The metabolic rate controls the rate at which sex hormones like progesterone and testosterone are produced by the body. Generally speaking, the higher your metabolic rate, the greater your sex hormone production. The primary hormone responsible for sex drive is testosterone in men and progesterone in women. Thus, higher metabolic rate yields increases in testosterone where it was previously lacking in men and greater production of progesterone in women—the hormone of female fertility (progesterone = pro-gestation-hormone). The net result in both men and women is greater sex drive and sexual performance, as well as ease of building muscle, greater leanness, enhanced athletic ability, and so on.

Redefining Fitness

(Dr. Garrett Smith)

Due to the thoroughly researched connection between excessive physical exercise and amenorrhea (the absence of a menstrual period in women of reproductive age), I wanted to go over a key term with multiple definitions: *fitness*. The original definition of *fitness* (circa 1580)—in the evolutionary biology context—is the ability to both survive *and* reproduce.

In recent times, the word *fitness* has been given additional definitions. One popular definition involves doing "work" within a given time frame, known to some as *work capacity*. The fittest people are often deemed the ones who can punish themselves and suffer the most through physical activities.

Here's the problem with embracing that definition. As Matt has pointed out, in women, a normal consequence of being subjected to long periods of high stress includes the menstrual cycle becoming more irregular or even disappearing altogether. Therefore, a woman who has reached a very high level of physical "fitness" in terms of work capacity through exercise training may actually be functionally infertile and completely lacking reproductive "fitness." The same is somewhat true in men who lose their libido and drive to pursue sex, even though these same men may be making enough sperm to still be technically fertile. It should be a given that if a man doesn't want to pursue sex and/or has trouble "getting it up," that's nearly on par with women who don't have a menstrual cycle in terms of outcome and reproductive "fitness."

In my opinion, infertility is one of the strongest indicators that something is very, very wrong in the body. A healthy woman in her childbearing years should be displaying every sign of fertility; her body shouldn't be abandoning the very process of fertility because it knows that it (and/or the fetus) could not survive the added stress of a pregnancy.

If you aren't familiar with it yet, ladies (and men who care about women's health), look up the condition *female athlete triad*, which is the sad combination of these three symptoms:

+ **Energy deficit and disordered eating**

+ **Menstrual disturbances and amenorrhea**

+ **Bone loss and osteoporosis**

Excessive stress—from overexercise combined with inadequate nutrition—causes negative hormonal shifts, which then leads to a disturbed menstrual cycle and bone loss.

Don't think that you'll get to avoid the bone loss part of the triad simply because you believe "strong is the new skinny" and you lift heavy weights regularly. In a study done to demonstrate the bone-building effects of oxytocin, it was shown that amenorrheic female athletes had lower nocturnal oxytocin secretion than female non-athletes of comparable body mass indexes (the infamous BMI that everyone loves to hate). The result was weaker bones in the amenorrheic female athletes, even though they were doing lots of weight-bearing exercise!

If your physical "fitness" sacrifices your reproductive "fitness," whatever you're doing is damaging your health, not helping it. By the time a woman's six-pack abs appear, her menstrual cycle has usually long since disappeared.

Fertility and Menstruation

Lack of a menstrual period, menstrual irregularity, PMS, and female infertility are most frequently caused by a lack of progesterone. During the first half of a woman's menstrual cycle (the first day of the period through roughly the fourteenth), estrogen dominates progesterone, meaning there is a much higher ratio of estrogen to progesterone than progesterone to estrogen in the body. This stifles the metabolism, which is why women's body temperatures are significantly lower during the first half of the cycle, sometimes by more than half a degree. The rise in progesterone during the second half of the cycle, however, stimulates ovulation, increases the sex drive, and stimulates vaginal lubrication and other pro-sex changes.

Metabolism-suppressing things like excess physical exercise; other forms of physical, psychological, and emotional stress; and calorie restriction cause many women to stop menstruating. Low progesterone is also partly responsible for menstrual symptoms like cramping and PMS.

By raising the metabolism, you can raise progesterone, which causes periods to return, menstrual symptoms to disappear, and fertility to improve.

High Cholesterol and High Triglycerides

Metabolism controls the rate at which LDL (also known as "bad cholesterol") is converted to progesterone and testosterone. Cholesterol in and of itself is a vital substance. To lower it with a drug, as millions of Americans are doing with statins, results in multiple symptoms, and most of them can be attributed to insufficient production of these vital hormones. The answer to high cholesterol is increasing the metabolic rate and turning "bad cholesterol" into these rejuvenating hormones associated with youth and disease resistance. A perfect example of this is a young man I worked with who dropped his "bad cholesterol" from 220 to 156, raised his "good cholesterol," and doubled his testosterone levels—all by simply raising his metabolic rate. The metabolic rate also controls the rate at which we burn, or oxidize, fuel. When the metabolic rate is high, triglycerides (blood fats) do not accumulate in the blood. High levels of triglycerides are a prominent risk factor for heart disease.

Heart Disease

The most successful doctor in the history of medicine at preventing heart disease was an American physician named Broda Barnes. Dr. Barnes made exhaustive and detailed records of his patients, cataloged them, and published the results in the 1970s. His patients experienced more than 90 percent fewer heart attacks than the general public at that time; only four of over two thousand patients had a heart attack, and each of these four had something out of the ordinary about them—one patient had only been seeing him for a few months, while another had just moved away and had discontinued his treatment. Dr. Barnes had this great success by making the metabolic rate the sole focus of his practice. He had patients keep track of their body temperatures to make sure that they maintained a youthful metabolic rate, thus avoiding diseases of the elderly. He treated countless other health problems using the same protocol. His book, *Solved: The Riddle of Heart Attacks,* was overlooked by the medical community already entrenched in an ineffective war on cholesterol. As a result, his theories have never been challenged on the scientific level, and his results have never been matched.

Cancer

Cancer is a disease of impaired cellular respiration. Many have theorized that the one consistent commonality among all forms of cancer is a lack of sufficient oxygen. When oxygen levels are too low, cells cannot burn glucose for fuel, causing the formation of cancer cells, which operate under a more primitive type of cell metabolism known as *anaerobic glycolysis* (which means the cells convert glucose to lactic acid). Estrogen, present in both men and women, is the primary antirespiratory hormone that chokes off the oxygen supply to cells. Estrogen is opposed by progesterone and testosterone, the hormones of youth, and, as we've discussed, the metabolic rate heavily influences how much of these hormones is produced. As metabolism falls in old age, cancer becomes much more likely. Our best defense is to keep metabolic rate as high as possible, which increases cellular activity, respiration, and cellular oxygenation. There is no better defense against cancer than optimizing a high metabolic rate.

These are just a few ways that the body is affected by the rate of metabolism. In addition, metabolism plays a big role in the rate of protein turnover and thus the rate of new tissue generation, which is how we heal wounds and build strong bones and teeth. It also figures prominently in blood sugar regulation. Metabolism lowers stress hormone production. It increases the potency of the immune system. It is involved in the production of red blood cells and other cells and tissues in general. Metabolism helps us to sleep longer and more deeply, as we did when we were kids. It controls our overall level of health, vitality, fertility, sex drive, strength, leanness, energy, and resistance to both degenerative and infectious disease. In short, a high metabolic rate represents youth!

In the next chapter I will show you how to interpret the signs your body gives you. The ability to read your metabolic biofeedback is perhaps even more important than the dietary recommendations to come. It's a good tool that will allow you to monitor your health throughout your life, and it's a great way of scoring the value of any health interventions you attempt.

Chapter 9

METABOLISM REPORT CARD

There are several signs, symptoms, expressions, and indicators of your metabolic state. Regardless of the diet you choose to follow, you can always monitor its impact on your body and hopefully experiment a little more freely to see what works. Without further ado, here are the most prominent barometers of good health. The eating, exercise, and other health practices you have adopted should always be judged based on success in these areas. Make acing this report card a priority!

1. Your waking temperature should be at least 98°F (36.7°C) every day. Higher temps are even better.

2. Your body temperature should rise even higher after meals and during the day, to 99°F (37.2°C) or above.

3. Your hands and feet should typically feel warm at normal room temperature.

4. You should experience a feeling of radiating plentiful body heat in general and dress lighter and feel as warm or warmer than those around you.

5. You should have fast-growing hair (on your head and body) and fingernails, with good shine to the hair and hardness to the nails.

6. You should have at least one (hopefully more) easy and large bowel movement per day that does not require straining or the use of laxatives, magnesium or vitamin C overdosing, or other bowel-moving crutches. Digestive troubles, such as irritable bowel

syndrome (IBS), stomach bloating after meals, excessive gas production, and heartburn, should be minimal or nonexistent.

7. You should urinate roughly once every four hours during the day, *never* at night, with no strong urges. The color should be yellow, never pale or clear.

8. You should be able to sleep through the night—a solid eight hours or more without waking.

9. If you are a premenopausal woman, you should have a regular menstrual cycle with normal flow and very few, if any, symptoms of PMS, cramping, bloating, and other common complications.

10. If you are a man, you should have full erections and good sex drive. Women should also feel pretty frisky and have good vaginal lubrication with strong sexual urges, particularly around the time of ovulation.

There are *dozens* more, but you'll drive yourself nuts trying to notice every tiny thing about your body. These are the basic barometers of good physical function that most deserve your attention. If there was an honorable mention, it would probably be moist skin, including on the hands and lower legs and feet, which often become dry when metabolism is reduced. Others include stable blood sugar, mood stability, good strength and muscle tone, and better than average resistance to colds, flu, and other common infections.

With these in mind, let's finally talk food!

Chapter 10
EAT FOR HEAT

What we're after here is pretty simple: Eat for heat. That is, you want to eat in a way that triggers what I commonly refer to as the "net warming effect." You want the combinations of food and fluids that you take in—and your daily diet as a whole—to trigger a noticeably greater production of internal heat. This should show up on a thermometer and in the way your body behaves: Your hands and feet should feel warmer, and you should feel warmer when the weather is cool—you should literally radiate body heat. The only time you should consider *not* eating for heat is in the peak of summer in a hot climate, when you are protecting yourself from heat stress. But even eating for heat when it's hot should simply trigger more sweating, allowing you to cool off.

Heat is not necessarily what we're really after—we're after health. But heat is a great and simple thing to focus on because internal heat represents a higher metabolic rate. This higher metabolic rate is what yields so many other health dividends.

This may seem complicated at first, but bear with me. It's really not. It seems appropriate though, given the equation theme, to give you a base equation from which we are working. For most people, getting the net warming effect from eating will be a matter of appropriately manipulating the following formula.

$$\text{Metabolic Increase} = \frac{\text{Calories} + \text{Carbohydrates} + \text{Salt}}{\text{Volume} + \text{Water Content}}$$

The primary warming substances are calories, carbohydrates, and salt. What determines whether they are warming or not generally depends on the volume and water content of the foods that contain those substances. In a nutshell, what we are talking about here is calorie density. The foods that have the highest ratio of calories to volume are the most warming, while the ones with the lowest ratio of calories to volume—like watermelon, with barely one hundred calories per pound—are the most cooling.

Most people are fearful of eating calorie-dense foods because most of our modern, iconic, "fattening" foods fit this description to the letter. The foods that would probably score the highest on the above equation would be pizza and potato chips. So before we continue, I ask you to suspend some of your preconceived notions about healthy nutrition. This is not a conversation about public health or ancestral diets. This is a conversation about *your* health and *your* individual, circumstantial needs. As I have said from the beginning, the diet that works today doesn't always work tomorrow. As you know, I am not advocating any particular diet here; my intention is to help you become aware of the powerful metabolic fine-tuning available to you right now.

Yes, you can overdo it on calorie-dense foods. Yes, it is about finding the right balance. If anything, you want to be eating the least calorie-dense foods *and still be achieving the desired results.* So maybe cancel that Domino's Pizza order for the moment.

Okay, back to our equation.

In essence, the more calories, carbohydrates, and salt *per bite* of the food, the more it is metabolically stimulating. Interestingly, the more you beat down your metabolism or get really stressed, the more you tend to crave these calorie-dense superstars. Similarly, if you do have a bite that's really packing some serious diesel, you'll go nuts on it—hence my inability to stop at one double-scoop cone when I had just overexercised myself to the point of mild impotence.

I hope that's a simple enough concept. Also note that the water content is a big factor in all this. Stuff yourself silly with Oreo cookies and pizza, but if you consume too many fluids with it, all bets are off. Proportions are what matters. A single slice of pizza with a few sips of root beer will typically raise metabolic rate noticeably. Eat an entire pizza with a gallon of water and you'll be just as freezing cold as if you inhaled an entire watermelon.

Easy, easy. Relax. I didn't mean to upset you by making mention of such villainous foods. Stay with me on this. We're actually going to talk about how to pursue this metabolism increase as cleanly and healthfully as possible.

First, let's talk about pee—my favorite subject!

Chapter 11
GIVE A HOOT, DON'T DILUTE!

Matt Stone

Every health advocate on earth seems to recommend drinking half your body weight in fluid ounces every day, meaning that if you weigh two hundred pounds, you would need to drink one hundred ounces, or about three quarts, per day. If they are too lazy to calculate and personalize it, they recommend drinking eight 8-ounce glasses of water. And the already-large quantity of water recommended seems to be increasing more and more. I see lots of people recommending the consumption of a gallon or more of water every day!

You've probably also heard the recommendation to "pee clear" coming from all sides. I am about to explain why all of this is nonsense.

For starters, no one on earth could ever tell you how much water you need to drink. Our hydration needs change hourly. Let's say it's the dead of winter and you don't do any exercise; you have a large smoothie for breakfast, followed by two big mugs of coffee midmorning, followed by a big, juicy salad with watermelon at lunch, and your only exercise is lifting a pencil. The prescription for eight 8-ounce glasses of water doesn't change. But what if you ate a big pile of salty sausage, cheesy eggs, and salty potatoes for breakfast and followed that with an hourlong jog in hundred-degree heat? Should you really be drinking the exact same amount of water in each case?

Exercise exertion, the kind and quantity of the food you eat, the time of year, and the temperature outside—all these things influence how much water you should drink. So how do you know if you are drinking too much or too little? It's not something, unfortunately, that you can keep track of mentally. I mean, if you're very thirsty, you know you should drink something. But the best way to determine hydration levels is by looking at your urine.

Yes, this is yet another great example of Paleo being *in you*. Thirst is a result of evolutionary fine-tuning and, as with most things having to do with the human body, instinct trumps the conscious mind. It certainly trumps a universal water prescription with little regard for situational variables.

That being said, hydration—specifically the concentration of your body fluids—is very important. But it's not what you think. We live in a dehydration-phobic society. And, yes, dehydration is dangerous; it will give you a headache and impair your athletic performance. But overhydration is also dangerous. In a world of swelling beverage sizes, smoothies and other blended concoctions, juices, coffee and tea, and overstated water prescriptions—people are drowning.

What's really going on is a continual dilution of our body fluids, and this lowers body temperature—metabolic rate. Most people who pay attention to the metabolic feedback I mentioned earlier will notice that excess fluid consumption and pale urine coincide with poorer function in all the major barometers of the metabolism report card.

Ever taste tears? Sweat? That's your body fluid—your extracellular fluid, to be exact—leaking out. It tastes salty, like seawater, because it *is* salty. The medical field considers perfect extracellular fluid to have nine grams of salt per liter. What do you think it does to your body when you take in several liters of water per day, eat a bunch of foods with a high water content, guzzle a big cup of coffee or three, never break a sweat, and maybe even eat a low-salt diet with that?

At best, it causes your body to work overtime to maintain homeostasis (the regulation of internal conditions to stabilize health, regardless of the outside changing conditions). At worst, it severely dilutes your body fluids, including your blood to some degree (in a condition known as *hyponatremia*), and generally wreaks havoc on your system. You would be amazed at how many people I come across who are suppressing their body temperature by multiple degrees. The repercussions of this include headaches, migraines, seizures, blurred vision, mood swings, heart palpitations, dizzy spells, *nocturia* (peeing excessively at night) and thus insomnia, and countless other obnoxious symptoms both minor and major. All of this by just drinking too much fluid in proportion to the food and salt they are eating.

The most worrisome symptom is dry mouth, which results from the activation of the stress system. Yes, it sounds crazy, but drinking too much can make your mouth dry as a desert, resulting in the consumption of even *more* fluid. This is about as effective as taking more showers for dry skin or putting water on dry lips to moisten them.

We could go into much greater detail about all this, but the solution is simple and a more appropriate thing to focus on. I find the best yardstick to get the body ideally hydrated is to simply turn all our focus on the urine.

Unless you are about to perform strenuous exercise out in the heat, your urine should *not* be clear. In fact, if an animal's urine falls below a certain concentration (measured by specific gravity or brix), veterinarians worry and assume the animal is sick. Urine should be yellow—not pale or clear, not dark or brown. Additionally, not only should it be yellow, but the color should remain consistent.

Groundbreaking stuff here!

While it may sound silly, for those who are chronically diluting their body fluids, this is a very powerful intervention and shouldn't be underestimated.

A good baseline or target for most people is to urinate roughly once every four hours during the day and never at night. At no point should there be a strong, sudden urge to urinate, either, which is usually an indicator of an acute surge in stress hormones. Stress hormones are diuretic in nature and tend to trigger a sense of urgency—even after having just urinated, or without any sense of pressure building in the bladder prior to a sudden need to urinate. This is why people have a tendency to urinate when they are frightened. You may have also noticed a tendency to urinate frequently after an intense argument or other acute stress. You will also likely experience more frequent urination with less fluid if you are doing something that is causing excessive stress in general, such as training too hard, working too much, or undereating.

One of the definitive symptoms of a low metabolism is excessive urination, for many reasons, the most prominent of which is probably the substantial rise in glucocorticoids and adrenaline in a stressful, reduced metabolic state. Check out this definitive statement from *The Biology of Human Starvation* by Ancel Keys: "Polyuria and nocturia have been reported by practically every observer of starvation conditions."

I was, of course, on the edge of my seat reading that one, as I had experienced all the symptoms discussed in the book when I was starving out in the backcountry. I found it really peculiar at the time, since I wasn't drinking much, but I was urinating incessantly, sometimes every ten minutes.

Now that I work with a number of people with eating disorders, as well as many health fanatics, vegans, carbophobes, hard exercisers, hypothyroidism sufferers, and others who have suppressed their metabolic rates, I see this theme repeated again and again. The physiology behind it, although I won't bore you with too much of it here, is quite fascinating.

There are a couple of theories. One is that stress makes the mouth dry, triggering an overconsumption of fluids, which in turn dilutes the body's fluids. The other is that increasing thirst is the body's clever way of purposely lowering core body temperature to reduce calorie burn. I'm not too sure about the second scenario, as this dilution of body fluids typically increases the desire for salty foods—a desperate attempt to compensate for the excess fluids consumed. This observation was also made during starvation experiments and reported by Keys: "Along with the increased water consumption, starving persons tend to have a marked salt hunger and will consume several times the normal quota of salt if it is available."

The good news is that by reconcentrating body fluids to a metabolically stimulating level, you can correct many of the conditions and symptoms discussed above. You do this simply by using the metabolism equation referenced earlier: Eat more calories, carbohydrates, and salt in proportion to fluids, and by *fluids* I mean fluids both naturally found in food and consumed as actual beverages.

Before we dig fully into what a prometabolism eating regimen might look like, here are some simple suggestions to keep in mind.

Whenever your urine becomes too pale or clear, you urinate several times in rapid succession, or you have a strong, sudden urge to urinate, *eat a dry, salty, carbohydrate-rich snack or meal as soon as possible.*

And lay off the fluids for at least an hour.

The objective here is to keep urine concentration—and thus the composition of your body fluids—as stable as possible. Maintaining consistency in the ratio of water to salt in your body fluids (carbohydrates are necessary for that to work properly, which is why all rehydration beverages, such as Pedialyte and Rehydran-N, contain both sodium *and* glucose) is not a panacea or cure-all. But it does take a tremendous load off your system, which is trying to regulate these things. When it comes to metabolic enhancement, helping your body maintain a healthy balance of certain essential substances is what makes the difference between making progress and not making progress.

Also, as I mentioned earlier, when your body gets into an overly diluted state, that prompts a surge of stress hormones. Combating the stress monster is all about minimizing the stress demand placed on your system, and avoiding dilution of your body fluids is a fantastic way to catch your stress spikes and quickly quiet them down. In other words, staying hydrated but not overhydrated is a powerful tool for reducing your stress exposure.

I wouldn't recommend being overly puritanical about your food choices in these emergency situations. In fact, if you want to shut down this stress cascade quickly, you shouldn't eat something that is going to sit in your stomach and be digested slowly, taking an eternity to actually get into your bloodstream, liver, and muscles. You want the fastest-absorbing carbohydrates, the ones that get into your bloodstream, liver, and muscles quickly. High-glycemic, starchy foods, like pretzels, popcorn, and potato chips, are actually preferable to "health" food in these situations.

If you are too busy to eat something substantial or even have a snack, consider combining a large spoonful of white sugar and salt and letting it dissolve under your tongue. Yes, white sugar! It actually has a medicinal effect in an acute stress situation. Adjust the flavor of the sugar-salt mixture to your liking, but keep it somewhere between a 4:1 and a 10:1 ratio of sugar to salt. This mixture is convenient and easy to carry around, and it's also good to keep by the bedside if you suffer from dreadful two to four a.m. wake-ups or multiple trips to the bathroom to pee in the night (stress hormones can rise to outrageously high levels at night if your metabolism is suppressed). This allows you to minimize disturbances in the night. You don't want to wake yourself up with a bunch of stumbling around in your kitchen or even chewing for that matter. The sugar-salt mixture often allows the nervous system to calm down enough for you to return to sleep and, if you're lucky, wake up in the morning not feeling like you've been hit by a bus.

So that's basically your acute intervention for what we'll call "crashes" from this point forward. Of course, the best strategy is to keep crashes from happening at all. And that's what we'll talk about in the next chapter.

Chapter 12
BALANCING THE EQUATION

By now, you should realize that this is far from a typical conversation about nutrition with definitive lists of "good" foods and "bad" foods. While you are undoubtedly skeptical at this point if you have anything going on in your skull that resembles brain-wave activity, I do want to remind you that the fundamentals of our physiology are far more important than the minutiae of nutrition. That's what most of the nutrition world seems to have upside down. I used to have it upside down, too. I'll lightly cover some of that before it's all said and done, but let's first continue to discuss some of the most useful and practical antistress, prometabolism interventions.

Body Temperature

We've talked about urination; now let's focus on your hands and feet. Start to become aware of the time of day that they tend to be coldest (this usually coincides with clearer urine and a sudden strong urge to pee). For most people, because of the normal human cortisol rhythm, which typically peaks in the morning, that time will fall somewhere between breakfast and lunch.

That's far from true for everyone, of course. Many people, particularly those who are not in peak condition, will see flip-flopped rhythms, with cortisol peaking at night rather than in the morning. At this time a sudden wave of coldness may strike, with strong cravings for dense calories (salt, carbs, and fat) and the onset of frequent urination.

Whatever your normal rhythm may be, pay attention to it and see if there is any consistency there. Once you've established the rhythm, it helps to play a little balancing game. If you have a tendency to crash out in the morning, you should plan on eating more calorie-dense foods—with more carbohydrates, more salt, and fewer fluids—in the morning. You may very well eat two-thirds of your total caloric intake for the day by one p.m. This will keep you warm and balanced with lower stress hormone exposure.

The rest of the day you can return to eating foods that have higher water content and drink more liberally. In other words, eat warming, metabolically stimulating foods when you are cold. After you have gotten your temperature up and climbed out of the dreary high-stress, low-metabolic state you experience during the first half of the day, spend the afternoon and evening maintaining that by eating less salt and concentrated calories and more of the iconic health foods: roots, fruits, beans, greens, salads, and soups.

At the other end of the spectrum, if you're one of those people who wear two pairs of socks to bed, you might fare better doing the opposite. Start the day eating cleaner and lighter, with foods like root vegetables, fruits, juices, smoothies, salads, and soups. Then eat a big, calorie-dense dinner and another calorie-dense bedtime snack. Never go to bed cold, hungry, or urinating frequently!

This may seem to be almost too insultingly simple to be effective, but do not discount its importance. Fundamentals rule! If you stop riding a big roller coaster up and down throughout the day and focus on staying in a balanced state of being from the time you wake up until the time you go to bed, it will pay off. The key, of course, is to keep at it. Consistency rules, too, especially if you can follow this regimen for many weeks and months.

The challenge for me in writing this is that I don't know you personally. You might be a person with a history of eating disorders and are therefore freezing-cold all day. In your case, the best way to balance your metabolism is to eat the most palatable and calorie-dense foods all day, with virtually no concern for the quality of those calories. The irony, of course, is that someone with eating disorder tendencies—after years of being overly focused on the minute details of food—is the least likely person to eat recreationally, as in eating whatever sounds the best at any given moment.

The point is that I can't make generalizations; nothing works for everyone. In the past, I have been roundly criticized for recommending foods like ice cream, pizza, cheeseburgers, chocolate, soft drinks, and potato chips, but I don't recommend those foods for everyone. They do, however, have a miraculous impact on someone who is really starving, because starving people typically do not have the digestive ability to eat fibrous, watery "health" foods. In such cases, calories matter above all else, and nothing packs it in like easily digestible calories found in the Standard American Diet.

Everything depends on the individual, and everything is on a spectrum of severity. People in the worst physical shape need the most calories, carbohydrates, and salt to heal. Those in pretty good shape can fully restore their metabolic rate to peak form without touching a single cookie. For that reason, all I ask is that you experiment freely and keep an open mind. Eat as nutritious a diet as you can while still nailing all the items on the Metabolism Report Card. If you can't do it eating "Paleo" or a strictly "clean," whole-foods diet, then eat all you want of fatty, salty foods without fear or remorse.

As psychologist Abraham Maslow noted sixty years ago, there is a hierarchy of needs, and there is nothing as stressful as failing to consume enough calories. In the realm of the health-conscious individual, undereating is a lot more common than overeating, which is why my general advice, in my near-decade of health research, has shifted from advocating dietary puritanism to encouraging a more relaxed, enjoyable, socially functional, and intuitive approach to nutrition.

Believe me, I have no love for Big Gulps, genetically modified food, feedlot meat, artificial flavorings, additives, MSG, hydrogenated oils, and pesticide-laced produce. I wish modern food wasn't completely inundated with that scary crap. But in real-world practice, for all the junk-food junkies in need of a clean diet to replace their regimen of pizza and ice cream, there are neurotic, clean-eating health Nazis or obsessive dieters in need of a slice of pizza and an ice cream cone to displace all the kale, brown rice, egg whites, and grass-fed beef that they are consuming. In the cod liver–scented bowels of the Internet, where most of my health information lurks, that statement holds even more truth.

Where do you fall on the metabolism spectrum? Only you can determine that, using some of the things discussed in this book, common sense, and some open-minded personal experimentation.

While focusing on calories is about as bland and boring and mundane as it gets—a distant leap from the excitement of mimicking the diet of isolated cave dwellers or megadosing on some mysterious nutrient found only in fish eyeballs or the nectar of an endangered Brazilian orchid—I can't help but redirect your attention away from all the noise and back to the basics. Again. Sigh.

Calories and Carbohydrates

Speaking of basics, let's talk calories. And carbs. Unlike the jillion other food-phobic cabbage munchers parading around the globe, I'm not worried about you eating too much. I'm worried about you eating too little—especially if you are intelligent enough to know that pursuing great strength and fitness and a vibrant, active life is an absolutely mandatory component to the health equation (and requires even more carbs and calories).

I want you to eat big and play hard (but smart and sustainable, as Garrett will inform you later) and to keep up with that consistently for years. To have the energy for exercise and to have the ability to recover from training hard, you need to keep your metabolism high, and to do that you need things like carbohydrates and calories. You need *lots* of those. Virtually no one has developed an elite physique or achieved great success in athletics without the consumption of copious amounts of carbohydrates and overall calories. If a few people managed to beat all odds and do it, that doesn't mean that you can, too, or that you won't break down into a quivering sludge of stressed-out, hypometabolic goop trying to imitate their diet and training regimen.

So how many calories and carbohydrates do you need? Like everything, it depends. It depends on your size, age, gender, and level of physical activity. At the very least, let's lay out some basic calculations on what the *minimum* amount should be.

First, estimate your total lean body mass in pounds as best you can—let's say it's the body weight you would have if you were lean enough to have visible abs. For me, that's about 195 pounds.

If you are an adult male under thirty years of age, multiply that weight by twenty. That's the minimum number of calories you should be eating per day.

If you are a female under thirty years of age, multiply that weight by eighteen. That's the minimum number of calories you should be eating per day.

If you are over age thirty, you have to factor in a slight, unavoidable decrease in basal metabolic rate that accompanies aging; it's just part of the natural wear and tear on our mitochondria. So if you are over the age of thirty, do the appropriate calculation for your gender and then subtract 1 percent for each year over thirty.

I'm thirty-five and male, so I would do the calculation as follows:

$$195 \times 20 = 3{,}900$$

Then I would subtract 5 percent, therefore multiplying 3,900 by .95, which equals 3,705.

If you were, say, a forty-eight-year-old female with an estimated visible-ab weight of 120 pounds, you would calculate your minimum calories like this:

$$120 \times 18 = 2{,}160$$

Adjusted for age: $2{,}160 \times .82 = 1{,}771$

For optimal performance, you should consume a diet that derives *at least* 50 percent of its energy from carbohydrates, and most people fare better metabolically and athletically with an even greater percentage of carbohydrates. So take your minimum calorie calculation and divide that in half to determine the number of carbohydrate-derived calories you need per day. For me, that would be:

$$3{,}705 / 2 = 1{,}852$$

Then divide that by four to determine the number of carbohydrate grams per day you need as a target minimum. For me that would be:

1,852 / 4 = 463 grams of carbohydrates daily

These are *minimums* to meet your optimal biological needs for good cellular energy production. *Minimums!* You'll need more if your physical activity is higher than average—perhaps much more. It's been found that in hard-training athletes, a minimum of ten to twelve grams of carbohydrates per kilogram of lean body weight in a twenty-four-hour period is required to fully restore muscle glycogen levels (carbohydrate stores). For someone my size, that could be over 1,000 grams of carbohydrates per day!

You don't have to count every calorie or carbohydrate you eat, of course, but if your metabolism is pretty low and you are suffering some of the signs of low metabolism, you need to maintain a surplus for weeks, sometimes months. Thus, it pays to become at least some-what calorie- and carbohydrate-aware. And yes, I said, *surplus*. For recovery, I have recommended multiplying your visible ab weight by twenty-three for males and twenty for females to yield even higher calorie intake until metabolism returns to normal.

Meal Frequency

Yes, another very exotic topic, I know.

Generally speaking, the lower a person's metabolic rate, the sooner the stress system becomes active during fasting. Someone with a very high metabolism can maintain homeostasis, has much bigger glycogen reserves, usually has a better-functioning liver, and can therefore maintain stable blood glucose levels for long periods. A very healthy person might be able to eat breakfast and go all day long consuming no other food, without changes in mood, fluctuations in energy, getting cold, urinating frequently, and so on. If your metabolic rate is lower, you might get cold hands and feet, get a weird taste in your mouth, and start to feel shaky within two hours of a meal. If this is the case, you will be far less able to go without food for extended periods without feeling the effects. So, generally speaking, the lower your metabolic rate, the more frequently you should eat.

After eating a meal, the body ramps up its oxidation of fuel for energy while also storing some of it in fat tissue and glycogen for later use. After a couple of hours, there is no fuel floating around and the body has to turn on hormones like cortisol, adrenaline, and glucagon to release stored energy. It's the rise in these hormones that elicits a stress event. That's normal human physiology to some extent. But the trouble starts if you are in really bad shape metabolically; then the stress response can be quite dramatic—at least that's been my experience working and communicating with people trying to improve their health.

Whether or not you experience any major negatives from going too long without food, I've come to believe that it's advantageous for healthy people to eat more frequently as opposed to less frequently. Stress hormones are catabolic, meaning they work to break down stored energy, including muscle tissue, when they are activated to supply energy. This is why bodybuilders looking to maintain the highest level of muscle mass in proportion to body fat tend to eat every two to three hours during the day; some of them even continue through the night in an effort to maintain every ounce of muscle mass possible while getting lean. The whole purpose of this type of eating is to minimize stress.

You don't necessarily have to adopt a strict bodybuilder meal schedule, but it illustrates the potential benefits of eating more frequently, particularly for someone who is recovering from being overstressed and underfed.

The density of your calories is another consideration when determining how often to eat. If you really want to eat a very clean diet—composed of natural, unprocessed, whole foods, which are invariably less palatable and calorie-dense than their refined counterparts—it's probably wise to eat more frequently. Since you are unlikely to eat as many calories at one sitting when eating clean, there's even more reason to spread your food out throughout the day into small, frequent meals. Potatoes, for example, are one of the more calorie-dense whole foods you can eat, and they only have 330 calories per pound.

Imagine trying to get 1,000 calories in a single sitting from just eating potatoes. Most people couldn't do it. I know I can't. Compare that with one of those tiny, 1,000-calorie containers of Häagen-Dazs ice cream. After two of those, I'm wondering what will be served next! This helps illustrate why eating foods with a low calorie density creates a need to eat more frequently in order to obtain an adequate number of total calories each day.

Do you need to eat a full meal every two to three hours? Probably not, although it's good to have a nice blend of the macronutrients each time you eat—as opposed to, say, just eating a piece of fruit for a snack, which is almost pure carbohydrate with little complementary protein, fat, or salt (and for those of you needing to raise your metabolic rate, salt should be considered an entire food group). Overall, the most convenient and realistic way to do it is to simply eat the standard three meals a day with a small snack between breakfast and lunch, another between lunch and dinner, and another before bed, if you need it. These snacks—if you are going to prioritize or emphasize a certain category of food—would be carbohydrates, both sugar (sweet-tasting foods like fruit or dried fruit) and starch (potatoes, beans, rice, corn, and so forth).

Since the whole point of eating these snacks is to quiet down the rise of stress hormones between meals, keep the primary metabolism-stimulating foods in the forefront of your mind. To help you remember these foods, as well as the concept, I call them the Antistress Ss: salt, sugar, and starch, with an honorable mention for saturated fat. Try to blend them together each time you eat.

As we discussed, snacks are most important when you feel the coldest and are the most in need of more food.

Salt

Before we move on, I'm sure you are still wondering exactly how much daily salt I'm talking about here. I'll bet you know the answer already—it depends!

It depends on how low your metabolism is and how diluted your fluids are at the beginning. There is no exact recommendation I can give you. I will say that any fears you have about consuming salt more liberally should be eased by the following points:

1. The most striking differences I have ever seen between death rates in a study group came in a recent study examining salt excretion rates (study title: "Fatal and Nonfatal Outcomes, Incidence of Hypertension, and Blood Pressure Changes in Relation to Urinary Sodium Excretion"). It is generally believed that salt excretion almost exactly matches intake, meaning you can tell how much salt a person eats based on how much salt passes in the urine. The more salt consumed, the more salt excreted. In the study, the group with the lowest excretion, and thus the lowest intake, had 500 percent more deaths than the group with the highest salt excretion and consumption. The in-between group fell right in the middle in terms of death rates. This study could very well be used to claim that salt is the single most protective substance ever found. I don't know if I would go that far—it's just one study—but it provides some pretty compelling evidence of the importance of salt.

2. When tracking the warmth of hands and feet and feelings of overall heat generation—as well as tracking actual body temperature with a thermometer—it becomes apparent that adding salt to the diet has an immediate temperature-boosting effect.

3. Most large academic inquiries into the relationship between salt intake and hypertension (the primary reason we are told to avoid salt) have found no such relationship. Other isolated studies show a weak correlation at best, with an increase of only a few points in blood pressure. Looking at all the data, it's clear that salt is a minor, if not completely insignificant, factor in blood pressure regulation.

4. Salt intake in some regions of Japan and China is as high as thirty grams per person per day. While you shouldn't ascribe some mythical perfect health to people in Asia just because obesity rates there are much lower than in the United States and Europe, they are clearly not dropping like flies from their high-salt diet. To give

you an example of how much salt thirty grams is, it is the equivalent of eating almost ten 7-ounce bags of barbecue potato chips every day. You probably couldn't eat that much salt if you tried. This may seem like an absurd amount, but keep in mind that medical doctors in America pump two or more liters of isotonic saline directly into the bloodstream of their patients every day to calm the nervous system, restore blood volume and good circulation, and so forth—and that's eighteen grams of salt, or roughly twice the average daily consumption of a typical American. So even your friendly doctor, who thinks salt is unhealthy, is saving lives daily by injecting massive amounts of it into people who aren't well!

I recommend erring on the side of too much salt rather than too little when starting out. You shouldn't salt foods to the point that they don't taste good, but you should have something noticeably but pleasantly salty showing up at every meal and snack. In severe cases, I sometimes recommend salting fruit and even drinks temporarily, but that's usually not necessary.

You should naturally find the right amount of salt for you. If you crave salt constantly or if you find putting plain salt directly on your tongue to be a tasty treat, you will probably reap exceptional benefits from eating a very salty diet.

A curious sidenote about salt: If you sprinkle it on the exterior of a potato chip or French fry, it tastes very salty. But it might surprise you to learn that chips and fries don't have anywhere near the salt content found in a juicy cheeseburger. A double cheeseburger at McDonald's has the same amount of salt as seven small orders of fries, and yet the fries actually *taste* saltier. Some foods absorb more salt than others and still taste good. Red meat and cheese seem to be the salt-spongiest of all foods; you can take in massive amounts of salt without their tasting too salty.

How much is too much? I can be a little more specific about this. The most obvious indications that you have overdone it include feeling as if you can hardly move—as if the force of gravity has doubled— your heart pounding loudly at night and keeping you awake (the sound of it seems deafening when your head is on your pillow), and restless legs combined with uncomfortably hot feet. Many of these symptoms seem to be related to blood volume expanding to dilute all the salt. When blood volume expands too much, the heart has to pump harder to circulate it. Plus, with all the extra blood, you really feel that hot blood pooling in your extremities. I can't go anywhere near super calorie-dense or salty foods late at night or my feet get so hot they feel as if they are burning.

So those are all a few basics, not so much about what you are eating specifically, but about when, how often, how much, and how to combine foods in a way to get the most metabolic mileage out of them. Mastering these fundamentals is far more important than your individual food choices, at least in my experience, but I will continue in the next chapter to give you some details that you are unlikely to have come across elsewhere.

Chapter 13

FATS, PROTEIN, AND CARBOHYDRATES

Hopefully by now you are thinking differently about nutrition. Maybe you're feeling a little freer to eat things you'd consigned to the no-no list. You don't have to be scared of fats or carbs for fear of developing heart disease or runaway diabetes. You don't have to be timid about meats or grains for fear of developing colon cancer or autoimmune disease. You don't even have to fear that wicked pint of ice cream. Ice cream may be exactly what you need at any given time in your life and on any given day. If your body is working pretty well, you are getting about as much as you can reasonably expect to get out of mindful nutrition and still fitting into today's modern world without being an extremist.

Because this is still something of a "Paleo" book, I will frame some of the following in a Paleo way. But please don't get the wrong idea: I have no interest in blindly mimicking the supposed diet of ancestral peoples with no regard for what science has already shown us.

When I first became a health researcher, I had a bias against science. I thought that a purely scientific approach to nutrition would never suffice. But I eventually discovered that much of my negative bias against science had nothing to do with science itself. It turns out that much of science, or what poses as science, that makes its way into the mainstream media has been hijacked by commercial interests, like pretty much everything else. However, underneath all the hype, fluff, fearmongering, political agendas, pharmaceutical interests, food industry motives, and bias lies plenty of useful and important information on the proper functioning of organisms, cells, and human beings.

Here are some basic aspects of nutrition that will help guide you toward better overall food choices on a daily basis.

Fats

Several decades ago *fat* became a nasty word. Researchers began attributing heart disease to the consumption of certain kinds of fat. Heart disease emerged from obscurity in the early twentieth century and continues to be the most frequent cause of death in industrialized nations today.

As anyone might do when looking to save millions of lives, the first heart disease researchers jumped to early conclusions based on an oversimplified understanding of the cause of coronary disease. They noticed that plaque in arteries contained large amounts of cholesterol. Plaque seemed to be what was blocking arteries and causing heart disease. They tested cholesterol levels in the blood and found that people with extremely high cholesterol levels had arteries that were more blocked than normal people. And since saturated fat seemed to increase blood cholesterol levels, at least temporarily, the researchers figured they had an open-and-shut case. *Artery-clogging saturated fat* instantly became a well-worn phrase in scientific circles, and this phrase is still abused more than a half-century later, despite dozens of discoveries that have since been made, showing that saturated fat doesn't have much to do with heart disease at all; that blocked arteries are just one *small* factor in the etiology of heart attacks; and that blood cholesterol levels have almost nothing to do with heart disease except in extreme cases (like familial hypercholesterolemia, which is inherited).

Anyway, that's just the *very* short version of my defense of saturated-fat consumption, which we now know has, if anything, a protective effect when it comes to heart disease and many other conditions because it protects and preserves our mitochondria. It does this primarily by defending against free radicals and one of the primary sources of free radicals, which is lipid peroxidation.

As most of you are probably aware, there are three primary classes of fats: saturated, monounsaturated, and polyunsaturated. Saturated-fat molecules are "saturated" with hydrogen ions, which makes them more solid at higher temperatures and, therefore, much more resistant to heat, light, and oxygen. Monounsaturated-fat molecules have an open space that is not bound with hydrogen ions, making them less stable and more liquid at normal temperature. Polyunsaturated-fat molecules have many open bonds, making them liquid at the coldest temperatures (even when water is below freezing) and very sensitive to heat, light, and air.

Nature operates in a very intricate way. The colder the climate, the more polyunsaturated fats there are in the food supply. Because of its properties, polyunsaturated fat is advantageous in cold climates. If a salmon had saturated fat in its tissues it would be as hard as a brick in cold water and unable to swim. Ever try to dig coconut oil out of a jar after it's been in the fridge? It's like trying to take scoops out of a bar of soap with a spoon, because it's 92 percent saturated fat.

But where do coconuts come from? Antarctica? Greenland? No, coconuts grow in the land of heat and sun, where saturated fats are highly protective. Fats generally fit the local climate as well as the seasons. In North America and Europe, polyunsaturated fats abound in the fall, when plants start making nuts and seeds that need to make it through the winter and germinate in cold soils in the spring. Nature is wicked smart and adaptable, too (kind of like me—um, right, guys? Guys?). Raising northerly crops in the tropics or raising pigs in hot weather will change their fat composition to something more saturated—protective against all that heat.

Those favoring Paleo diets make a strong pitch that grains and dairy products are modern inventions that humans have failed to adapt to eating (even though there is abundant evidence we have!). In reality, science points to the actual problem, which is that we have messed with the fats in our food supply, a fact that is central to the wave of diseases we are now experiencing in the modern world. Most of those diseases are known to be inflammatory and oxidative at their core, which makes polyunsaturated fat the most likely culprit on both fronts. This wave of inflammation is perhaps what is increasing sensitivities to Paleo-maligned foods like beans, grains, nightshade vegetables, and dairy products. Food allergies and sensitivities are almost certainly not caused by our failure to properly evolve. They are more likely caused by the way humans have violated the laws of nature with the major overhaul in the dietary fats we have been consuming over the past century.

I like to pinpoint root causes, and it never made much sense to me that brand-new diseases that exploded during the twentieth century could be linked to dietary changes that took place ten thousand years ago. It made a lot more sense to examine what changed immediately prior to the current epidemics of obesity, cancer, diabetes, heart disease, autoimmune disease, asthma, allergies, and so on—all of which began to increase in the early 1900s. And the biggest dietary shift since then has been the development and mass adoption of seed and vegetable oils.

Vegetable and seed oils are made from things like soy, corn, safflower, sunflower, cottonseed, grapeseed, canola, peanuts, and so forth. They are the oils used in nearly every modern restaurant, every packaged food, and every salad dressing, and they were scarcely used prior to 1900. At that time, people used butter, lard, beef tallow, olive oil, and coconut oil in their cooking. And, of course, everyone consumed whole milk and full-fat products.

Take a look at this U.S. government data on changes to the American diet between 1909 and 1999:

+ Consumption of whole milk dropped 49.8 percent

+ Consumption of skim milk increased 57.8 percent

+ Consumption of butter dropped 72.2 percent

+ Consumption of margarine increased 800 percent

+ Consumption of lard and tallow dropped 50 percent

+ Consumption of salad and cooking oil increased 1,450 percent

Note the massive displacement of saturated fats (butter, lard, tallow, and whole milk are mostly composed of saturated and monounsaturated fats) and the rise of products derived from vegetable oils (which have mostly polyunsaturated fats). This was an economically driven change as big-business tycoons found novel ways to create products to compete with traditional household fats and oils. Fast-forward to the twenty-first century and it's easy to retrace the economic origins of the saturated-fat scare, the cholesterol-lowering medication boom, and more. The U.S. government even began subsidizing the production of soy, corn, and other big cash crops for conversion into cheap oils and other by-products that now make up a considerable portion of the American diet. These oils have gone beyond the household and worked their way into nearly every mass-produced food product and restaurant meal, leading to larger profit margins for all who use them.

The purported health advantage of these vegetable oils is that they reduce cholesterol, so naturally doctors jumped all over them. At this point, even if the original recommendations to avoid saturated fat were an honest scientific mistake, you can be sure that the food and restaurant industries are not going to give up one of their top moneymakers anytime soon. And they have big allies in the medical community and the pharmaceutical industry, which make billions off cholesterol-lowering drugs. The message won't change because the financial well-being of so many industries depends on vegetable oil and the outdated idea that it wards off the cholesterol bogeyman. Contemporary nutritional, agricultural, medical, and pharmaceutical industries took a radical turn when vegetable oils were created. Now, genuine science faces an extremely difficult struggle against the vegetable oil–adoring, cholesterol-fearing stance of the world's biggest financial powers.

Okay, I'll quiet down my inner Alex Jones now.

"Pipe down, Alex! Go clean up your room. Ron Paul's coming over for dinner and you don't want him seeing this mess! That's right. Put all your American Eagle Silver coins back under your bed. You can play with them again tomorrow."

There, that's better. Let's move on to the specifics of how the fats in vegetable and seed oils hurt us. We now know that the type of fat found abundantly in these oils (linoleic acid primarily) plays a direct role in the production of an entire class of pro-inflammatory molecules. We also know that polyunsaturated fats are more unstable than saturated; they oxidize much faster on the shelf, in the frying pan, and in our bodies. We are therefore exposing ourselves to a very large load of free-radical oxidation when we consume polyunsaturated fats.

Ever heard of antioxidants? Know why they are good for you? Know why they are found to be protective against most degenerative diseases? It's because they work to combat all the oxidants that we are taking in and producing when each and every one of our cells is filled with (confirmed to be filled with—this is not just speculation) polyunsaturated fats.

Just about all degenerative diseases have three things in common:

1. Inflammation

2. Free-radical damage

3. Decreased energy production (i.e., decreased mitochondrial respiration and ATP production—better known as a reduced metabolic rate)

The polyunsaturated fats we now consume in almost everything we eat at every meal, to a degree that could never be replicated in nature (these fats are only found seasonally in certain climates), represent the most significant dietary change in history. There have been many changes throughout history—some good for our health and some not so good—but this is the mother lode.

It's the most significant because the type of polyunsaturated fat found in these oils and products plays a direct role in worsening each of the three commonalities of degenerative disease, present in everything from diabetes to asthma to Alzheimer's to heart disease. Inflammation, free-radical damage, and decreased metabolic rate are all exacerbated by excess consumption of these fats. They also go by the names *linoleic acid* or *omega-6 fatty acids;* they are more or less the antithesis of the omega-3 fats you've heard so many good things about.

Unfortunately, the story gets worse. We also create this type of fat in much of our farm-raised meat, eggs, and fish. We do this by feeding large quantities of corn and soy to livestock. While this has little effect on ruminant animals like cows and sheep, who convert everything they eat to mostly saturated and monounsaturated fats in their bellies, it has a very powerful impact on pork, poultry, and farmed fish; much like ours, their tissues are a direct reflection of the fatty acid composition of their diets.

"What are we serving tonight? Chicken or . . . chicken?" —Tom Callahan, Jr., aka Tommy Boy

Here's another thing that increased between 1909 and 1999: poultry consumption, by 278 percent. So we are not only feeding more corn and soy to chickens, but we are also eating far more chicken. Pork consumption has remained about the same, however, and it is still consumed in the highest quantities in the American South and Polynesia, places with some of the poorest health statistics in the world.

Not to get too nerdy on you, but the reason linoleic acid (LA) from vegetable and seed oils correlates so strongly with inflammation is the end product it leads to after going through a chain of physiological processes in the body. After passing through a few steps, the fatty acid arachidonic acid (AA) is formed. The more LA in the diet of humans, pigs, chickens, and farmed fish, the more AA you can expect to find in the cells and tissues of that animal. Inflammation seems to be more or less directly related to the cellular concentrations of AA. Floyd Chilton of Wake Forest University has done research regarding the connection between arachidonic acid and inflammatory diseases, asthma in particular:

> . . . Research has proven that a high–AA diet has the potential actually to change normal immune responses to abnormal, exaggerated ones. A study carried out in 1997 by Dr. Darshan S. Kelley and colleagues at the Western Human Nutrition Research Center in California showed that people on high–AA diets generated four times as many inflammatory cells after a flu vaccination as people on low–AA diets.

So what's a high-AA diet? It's one that contains the meat of factory-raised pigs and poultry, as well as factory-farmed eggs and farmed fish. In fact, the biggest dietary sources of AA are the fattier portions of those foods.

The long story short here: Humans have seriously meddled with the food supply in a biologically significant way. As you have probably heard elsewhere, these changes have resulted in a huge increase in the proportions of omega-6 to omega-3 in our cells, tissues, fat, and even breast milk—more specifically, the ratio of AA to EPA (eicosapentaenoic acid, a type of long-chain omega-3 found in greatest concentration in all those fish oils you've been gagging down).

While I think it's unreasonable to expect anyone to strictly avoid any kind of food entirely, this is worth bringing to your attention. It's also worth noting that the problem isn't a lack of omega-3s in the diet; the amount of omega-3 fatty acids in tissues and breast milk appears to have remained consistent for well over half a century. (In fact, evidence is building that we are not meant to take in huge quantities of omega-3s, and we may be overdosing on fish oil.) Rather, we should stop eating so much effing LA and AA!

Again, don't get extreme with this. It takes a long time to bring fatty acids back into balance—sometimes many years. Don't forget that we are combating a multigenerational accumulation of these fats in our bodies. So reduce your consumption of these types of fats in a moderate and sustainable way. Anything you do will have a positive impact and, as I hope you've gathered by now, long-term practicality and effectiveness are best achieved with modest interventions.

Here are a few simple tips regarding the consumption of fats. They are all recommendations, not commandments.

1. Choose red meat or wild-caught fish and seafood over pork and poultry.

2. If you do occasionally eat pork (I don't), choose lean cuts like loin and tenderloin; bacon, sausage, and ribs contain the bulk of the AA found in pork.

3. When you eat poultry, don't eat the skin (or if you do, eat it only on occasion).

4. Don't eat whole eggs every day; try them once or twice a week or as an ingredient in your baked goods, which is how I consume most of my eggs. If you go to great lengths to obtain eggs from wild-fed, pastured hens, you can probably consume eggs more frequently, as the fats in the yolks are much more balanced.

5. Avoid deep-fried foods at restaurants.

6. Use butter, ghee (clarified butter), coconut oil, and macadamia nut oil as your household cooking and salad oils. Olive oil is okay but not ideal, containing about 10 percent linoleic acid, which is much less than the oils from corn, soy, canola, cottonseed, sunflower, and company.

7. Choose macadamia nuts over other types of nuts and seeds, like peanuts, sunflower seeds, pumpkin seeds, almonds, pecans, walnuts, and others, all of which are very high in polyunsaturated fat.

8. Reduce your consumption of high-fat packaged foods like chips and cookies; low-fat packaged foods like breakfast cereals, saltines, and pretzels are fine.

9. Use sour cream instead of mayonnaise in recipes that call for mayonnaise.

10. Don't eat any commercial salad dressings except those made with olive oil. Make your own creamy dressings with a sour cream base or vinaigrettes made with macadamia nut oil.

There are others, but if this list got any longer you probably wouldn't remember any of them!

Contrary to mainstream opinion, the best place to get your fats is actually from saturated fats—the more saturated the better. The most saturated fats come from coconut, cocoa butter (chocolate), red meat, and dairy fat. That doesn't mean that they are medicinal and that the more of them you eat the better. Our cells generally produce energy a lot more efficiently, with more carbon dioxide production as a bonus (which is very de-stressing and stimulating to the metabolism), when carbohydrates provide the bulk of our dietary energy. So it's not a matter of "the more the better" when it comes to saturated fats; just go easy on unsaturated oils, nuts and seeds, and high-AA meats, and replace them with more saturated fats. You probably won't feel any amazing differences in the short term, but this kind of dietary change is a very positive investment in your long-term health.

Protein

Up until this point, I've barely mentioned protein. Fact of the matter is, if you are eating plenty of food, and plenty of carbohydrates, it's virtually impossible to fail to meet your daily protein needs unless you are a vegan or hard-training athlete.

With all the positive information and products out there glorifying protein, and the rest of the nutrition world talking smack about either carbs or fats, protein often gets a better reputation than it deserves.

Protein is essential to the body, and health quickly deteriorates when the body loses muscle mass from inadequate protein consumption, but there are some subtleties to protein consumption that don't get talked about often.

Protein is made up of chains of amino acids. While we need those amino acids, they are not all created equal. If we take a look at protein from the Paleo point of view, it becomes evident that we don't eat the richest sources of protein—protein from animal products—in the same way as was traditionally practiced. Today, we mostly eat the tender cuts of muscle meat and the fleshy parts of fish. Other health-focused people supplement this further with whey-based protein shakes and who knows what else in order to obtain protein in a "more the better" type of fashion.

But in most traditional cultures, and even in traditional cooking, the *whole animal* was used. Bones, skin, head, hooves, feet, organ meats, and bone marrow—all were consumed in addition to the muscle meats. Wild meats are also much richer in connective tissues and are quite leathery compared to the filet mignons and rib eyes on the menu at your favorite restaurant. Many experts have highlighted the fact that organ meats are the most nutritious parts of an animal and probably should be eaten on occasion, and I don't disagree. But equally, if not more significantly, the amino acid profiles of muscle meat are very different from the amino acid profiles of bones and connective tissues. As we dive deeper into this discussion, you'll see that eating only the tender parts of an animal leads to an unbalanced protein intake.

The fleshy parts of fish and animals tend to be very rich in amino acids like cysteine, methionine, and tryptophan—amino acids that have been found to have numerous negative biological effects. Diets that restrict methionine to a significant degree appear to prolong life span as much or more than any other known dietary intervention. A high consumption of cysteine (and methionine) has a tendency to raise homocysteine levels in the blood, a by-product of a metabolic process called the *methylation cycle*. According to Kilmer McCully of Harvard University, elevated homocysteine levels are a strong risk factor for heart disease. Tryptophan, a precursor to the formation of serotonin (almost criminally anointed the "happy chemical"), raises blood pressure and increases inflammation, among other negative effects.

On the other side of the fence, all the protein bound in the connective tissues, skin, bones, and so on that are too often discarded in today's diet, contain a very different amino acid profile—one that is very anti-inflammatory in nature. This is collagen, also referred to as gelatin—a substance worshipped in traditional cookery and cultures in the form of meat stocks, gelatinous sauces, and all those nice things.

This may sound quite complicated, but it's really not. The practical, everyday approach to fixing this imbalance is easy: Get more protein from plants and gelatin, and go easy on the muscle meat.

The three most significant ways to obtain more gelatin are the following:

1. Make homemade, bone-based meat stocks and sauces (a massive chore).

2. Buy cuts of meat with more bone and connective tissue, like beef or lamb shanks, oxtail, short ribs, whole fish with head and

bones, and whole birds (including the feet if you can get them), and slow-cook them to tenderize and extract the gelatin.

3. Buy a gelatin powder (the best beef gelatin and collagen hydrolysate products are from Great Lakes Gelatin). Add a couple of tablespoons to your diet daily, extra with meat and fish dishes to offset the amino acids in them. It's great in soups or broths, or it can be added to milk, juice, and other drinks, hot or cold. It can also be used to make gelatin desserts like fruit-juice Jell-O, marshmallows, candies, or panna cotta. This is the only way, in my experience, that we can get enough gelatin in our diet to notice its benefits.

And don't forget that plant foods have protein, too. While the protein in grains, beans, legumes, tubers, vegetables, and fruit is not as useful to the body as that found in eggs, milk, fish, and meat, there is still a decent amount in there. Most plant foods, like the ones I just listed, will be 10 percent protein when averaged together. If you are meeting the daily carbohydrate requirements that I laid out earlier and adding some gelatin to your diet, you will certainly get an adequate amount of protein.

While you won't catch me on a vegan or vegetarian diet any time soon (been there, done that), I don't want you thinking that there is some obligatory need for a big hunk of meat at every sitting. There simply isn't, and it's probably disadvantageous to consume more protein than you need. If your calorie and carbohydrate intake is adequate—both of which have a pronounced protein-sparing effect (meaning, more or less, that you use the protein you eat a lot more efficiently)—the need for protein falls right around one gram per kilogram of lean body weight per day, and certainly no more than one gram per pound of lean body weight per day.

You can even build muscle on this intake, and you'll probably do so more successfully than if you try to eat your body weight in protein every day. That's because protein suppresses appetite and requires more calories to digest, and calorie intake is by far the most important factor when it comes to growing new muscle tissue. After all, the time when we grow new lean tissue the fastest is on breast milk, which is only 6–7 percent protein by percentage of overall energy consumption. In our calorie-phobic society, protein is the hero because it suppresses appetite and more calories are burned during digestion. But I'm looking at the big picture and, as far as long-term health goes, eating a lot to support a high metabolism and keeping your protein intake moderate reduces inflammation and likelihood of injury, while allowing you to train harder and recover faster.

Carbohydrates

Here we are at what I'm sure will be the most controversial and criticized part of this book among the Paleo community: carbs.

Pretty much everything you've heard about carbs being the root of all evil is a breathtakingly beautiful example of an oversimplified, sciencey-sounding, but totally false theory. Just about every detail of the low-carb sermon that you've heard in books and on websites is simply not true. From "sugar causes cancer" to "carbs raise insulin and cause obesity and diabetes"—it's all pretty laughable.

Going back to some Paleo thinking, how many carbohydrates did our ancestors eat? Humans that lived in the tropics obviously ate quite a bit. We are the only primate species that managed to escape the Tropics of Capricorn and Cancer, and most humans today still live pretty close to the equator.

Almost all other primates still live in very tropical climates and a very high percentage of them subsist on a fruit-based diet, with 70–90 percent of their calories supplied from carbohydrates. Most of the earth's population continues to derive 70 percent or more of their dietary energy from carbohydrates, including the people who live in Africa and Asia, where population density is highest. There are hunter-gatherer societies still in existence—the Kitavans, for example—who continue to eat high-carbohydrate diets. I should add that pretty much any successful competitive athlete eats in a similar fashion.

So I'm going to go out on a limb and say that carbohydrates are safe. They're actually preferable when compared to other energy sources. And when you add in regular physical activity, which we obviously consider a mandatory part of the equation, then a high-carb diet has even more advantages. Whatever you can do on a low-carb diet, you can probably do better on a high-carb diet. The naturally contrary parts of me led me to believe otherwise for a time, but my body, after years of carbohydrate restriction, told a different story—and many others corroborated my experience. I wanted to believe that fat was some undiscovered optimal fuel source and ate 300 grams of it per day on average for several years, but it just isn't.

The big issue in the pro-carb world right now involves finding the best source. Is it best to get them from simple sugars (things like fruit) or starches (grains, tubers, and legumes)? There is no clear answer, but I tend to think that nearly everyone does better with some of both—if for no other reason than that when you have variety, food is more palatable and you eat more of it!

Nutritious, unrefined carbohydrates like fruit, potatoes, sweet potatoes, yams, and other root vegetables are a great foundation for most diets. Whole grains, as well as beans and legumes, can trigger digestive distress for a lot more people and, if that's the case for you, it's fine to avoid them.

Many nutrients are removed during the refining process of grains like white rice and white flour, but as long as your diet is not solely composed of these foods and you are getting plenty of nutrition over-all, it's okay to eat a substantial amount of them. Lost nutrients aside, they are a heck of a lot easier to digest than whole grains, and refining removes a great deal of the linoleic acid found in the whole grain as well. In the real world it's tough for a person who is exercising regu-larly to meet the necessary daily carbohydrate quotas without eating at least a little refined grain.

Other sources of carbohydrates that you may do really well with, especially if your metabolism is low coming into this, are the super-concentrated sources of sugar—maple syrup, blackstrap molasses (perhaps the most mineral-dense food on earth), honey, date sugar, coconut sugar, fruit juice, dried fruit, and even (gasp!) some white sugar.

Whatever you've heard, and despite what you might have experienced by eating lots of carbohydrates in the past, I think you'll be pleasantly surprised by the results of eating this way. Just make sure it is in conjunction with progressive exercise, good sleep, stress reduction, reasonable quantities of fat, balanced amino acids, and a big reduction in dietary linoleic acid and arachidonic acid. But give your body adequate time to adjust and don't panic when you get some pimples, retain a little water, or feel a little bloated for the first few weeks. That's just what happens when your body adjusts to this new and dramatic way of eating.

Sugar Strength

Dr. Garrett Smith

Many people will not want to add carbohydrates to their diet because they say their blood glucose numbers will "go crazy," along with a host of other symptoms. Often these folks have been doing low-carbohydrate dieting for so long that the addition of any carb to their system throws their delicate, fully stress-hormone-mediated state of homeostasis completely out of whack. Or some just get a couple of zits, a little bloating, and gain a couple pounds and immediately run back to their old methods. Running away from the solution takes you back to the problem.

I like to use the example of strength training in this case. If you avoid like the plague lifting anything heavy—due to an irrational fear of injury and muscle damage—it would be very likely that over time you would get weaker, correct? Making you less "tolerant" of lifting heavy things, yes? "Yeah, yeah," you say, "get to the point."

After eventually realizing just how weak you've become by avoiding lifting anything and accepting that there is a small amount of risk inherent in any type of exercise, you then decide to start strength training because the benefits outweigh the risks. What happens then? In addition to being weak and not good at it, you get *sore* and it *hurts*. This lasts at least a couple of days, maybe even up to a week. It is not pleasant, yet you have learned and accepted that to get what you want, an initial period of discomfort must be endured. It was your choice initially to stop lifting, and there is a price to be paid when you get back into it. You also know that the soreness will decrease over time and you'll receive the reward of stronger muscles, bones, tendons, heart, and so on.

Now, let's apply that same idea to carbohydrate metabolism. You chose at some point to go low-carb. If you were successful in avoiding carbohydrates for long periods—prompted by bloggers with irrational fears and misunderstandings of how the body really works—wouldn't it be likely that over time your body's carbohydrate metabolism would get *weaker* and you would become less tolerant of sugars and starches?

The reality is that when you reintroduce sugars and starches to your diet, you will likely have an initial period of discomfort and some associated symptoms. This is not the "carb flu" or other nonsense propagated by the carbophobes. If and when you realize that your symptoms are due to your body having grown weak in its sugar metabolism over time, that eating more carbohydrates is actually the only way out of the cycle, and that change by its very nature is uncomfortable, you will be able to cope more easily with any minor symptoms that pop up during the early stages of metabolism rehab.

Break the cycle. Stop the insanity. Suck it up, buttercup. Many other clichés will work here, too. I hope to see you on the other side!

Carbohydrates are even more important before, during, and after exercise. This is when you need to *really* make an effort to carb up and deliberately consume fast-absorbing carbohydrates that have little or no fiber, such as the quickly absorbed, glucose-based workout drinks that contain things like maltodextrin and dextrose. The faster carbohydrates get into your system after a workout, the faster you start recovering and the more productive your exercise regimen will be long term. The postworkout period is a pivotal time when your body's stress system is going wild.

Antimetabolism Foods

As a last tidbit, because it doesn't really fit anywhere else or deserve its own chapter, there are some foods that you shouldn't consume in excess because they contain antithyroid compounds. Notice that I didn't say you should fear them or never eat them because they are "bad." But there are a lot of health fanatics misguidedly and excessively consuming these foods, thanks to popular nutrition authors like Joel Fuhrman.

Those foods are beans and legumes, as well as cruciferous vegetables, which include kale and kale juice, collard greens, arugula, watercress, bok choy, cabbage, broccoli, and cauliflower. Cooking helps to reduce the thyroid-interfering properties of cruciferous vegetables, but health nerds with a "more the better" approach often make the mistake of eating or consuming the raw juice of crucifers.

Eat some of these types of foods when you desire them, sure, in reasonable amounts. But I would caution against basing your whole diet on beans, lentils, soy, and cruciferous vegetables.

Chapter 14

WHAT A HEALTHY DIET LOOKS LIKE

Oh, I see you there, rubbing your hands together, eager to hear exactly what you are supposed to eat. You want specifics. You want a thirty-day meal plan. "Just tell us what to do, guys!"

Sorry, basics again. You can go back to sleep.

The most important thing about eating has nothing to do with whether a caveman ate it or even how you fill *your plate*—with potatoes or fruit, yams or grains, meat or fish or whatever. It is that you are eating food off *your plate*. You own that plate. It sits in your house, where you are eating food that you bought or grew, that you made in your oven, using your fork, your spoon, and your knife.

If you want to get as much out of your nutritional choices as possible, in a realistic and sustainable way, you should habitually cook and eat most of your food at home on your plates, or out of food containers that you own and put in your dishwasher at the end of the day. You should also be sitting down when you eat them, preferably at a table and not in bed or behind the wheel of a car or in front of your computer screen.

Hey, I'm no stranger to eating at restaurants or grabbing food on the run. I wouldn't discourage anyone from dining out on a regular basis, and grabbing a quick snack is certainly better than not eating at all. Nutrition isn't everything there is to life. However, if you want to eat a good diet consistently and reap the rewards from maintaining a healthy diet for years and decades, it's best to get in the habit of participating in the preparation of your own food and eating mindfully. Overall, the most important piece of advice anyone can give you is to keep your food in your hands and not place it in the hands of others who are looking to cut costs and spice up cheap ingredients for profit.

That also means that most of your food should be prepared from simple and mostly fresh ingredients that are not packaged and ready to eat. We all know this; it's common sense. Yet commonsense wisdom is powerful—far more powerful than the obscure telomere research awaiting you on the Internet or the new gadget in a late-night infomercial.

Aside from that, eat a wide variety of foods. Meals today are increasingly incomplete—a smoothie is not a meal; it's a beverage. If I served that to my girlfriend's eight-year-old kid and called it "breakfast," I might get a crotch full of fast-moving fist. A salad is not a meal—it's hardly food at all! Try to work several components into your meals, including something sweet, something starchy, something salty, and something hearty. Your meals will be more enjoyable and more satiating. They will keep your mood, energy, and metabolism stabilized, which will keep you from getting ravenous and pigging out on packaged junk.

Chapter 15
BODY FAT

Contrary to almost everything you have heard, weight is not a good predictor of health. In fact, a moderately active larger person is likely to be far healthier than someone who is svelte but sedentary. Moreover, the efforts of Americans to make themselves thin through dieting and drugs are a major cause of both "overweight" and the ill health that is wrongly ascribed to it. In other words, America's war on fat is actually helping cause the very diseases it is supposed to cure.

There is no good evidence that significant long-term weight loss is beneficial to health, and a great deal of evidence that short-term weight loss followed by weight regain (the pattern followed by almost all dieters) is medically harmful. Indeed, frequent dieting is perhaps the single best predictor of future weight gain.

—Paul Campos, *The Obesity Myth*

No twenty-first-century health book would be complete without a little discussion about body fat, right? That's all anyone in this insane culture seems to care about these days. Virtually every magazine promises "7-minute abs!" or has the last word on belly fat. And, as you've read in this book so far about high calorie intake, calorie-dense foods, and getting more rest, I suspect this sounds to you like a perfect recipe for becoming a blob.

The people who need this information the most are chronic dieters and food restrictors. That's because these are the people who are the most primed for fat storage when they begin feeding themselves properly and getting the rest they need to improve metabolism and overcome stress-induced health problems. This will be scary to those people because, yes, gaining fat in the short-term is a strong possibility, but it's a *good thing*! The hormone leptin, which increases as fat tissue increases, is the primary hormone signaling the hypothalamus to increase the metabolic rate of each and every cell in the body. Making this hormone surge is one of the most therapeutic things a sick person can do; it is the primary driver of the whole rebuilding and recovery process.

What I recommend you do—thin or fat—is to get to the point where you are maintaining a steady weight while doing as much exercise as you desire and no more, and eating as much food as you desire and no less. With that formula, you will end the fight and begin allowing your body to regulate its fat levels.

It's what I like to call "fat-proofing." Yes, of course you may gain some fat in the short term when you stop playing the silly calories-in, calories-out game on a conscious level. But in the long term, you will earn great dividends for your health and your body composition.

We now know, both experientially and scientifically, that creating a conscious calorie deficit—what is called "intentional weight loss"—is extremely harmful, putting one at much greater risk of developing major, long-term health problems (despite temporary improvements in blood lipids and other markers). But it also worsens body composition. *Body composition* is a term referring to the relative amounts of body fat and lean tissue like bones, organs, and muscles. From an aesthetic standpoint, most people look their best when body fat percentage is low (although when forcing fat off their bodies they may look nice but be a total metabolic wreck underneath) and lean tissue is high. During intentional calorie deprivation, lean tissue atrophies along with lost pounds of fat, and when weight is regained, as inevitably happens in 95–99 percent of individuals, fat accumulates much faster than lean tissue. The end result? Even if your weight returns to the exact same place in terms of the number on the scale, you look worse, with less muscle tissue and more body fat.

In calorie-restriction experiments carried out by Ancel Keys during World War II, thirty-two subjects regained their abdominal fat the fastest—regaining 101 percent of the loss in their waist measurements in just twelve weeks—yet their arms and legs were still tiny and weak. By the time they had restored the lost lean tissue in their arms, legs, and chests, they had managed to reach body fat levels 40 percent higher than at the start of the experiment. It wasn't eating carbs or fats or too many calories, or having too few CrossFit sessions, that made them fat; what made them fat was first eating less than 2,000 calories per day for twenty-four weeks, then returning to their normal habits of eating whatever they wanted, whenever they wanted. They didn't get fat eating whatever they wanted before.

They needed a harsh diet first to make that possible. Repeated dieting is the ultimate fat on-switch.

Instead of repeatedly losing fat and muscle and then regaining fat without the muscle again and again and again, as people are doing in the modern world, I recommend the opposite approach—reverse yo-yo dieting, in a sense. Eat a lot, sleep a lot, do some resistance exercise, gain some muscle, and then eat according to your appetite in a sustainable way and without long-term harsh dietary restrictions. If the fat still isn't coming off, creating a tiny intentional calorie deficit by increasing your physical activity levels or eating a lighter dinner may help. Even this slight change still comes with the risk of shutting down your metabolic rate and is not something I typically advise. Taking more extreme action is even more dangerous.

The long-term result of eating well and avoiding diets like the plague will be muscle gained in proportion to body fat. All the while, you will be maintaining a high metabolic rate and reaping all the health benefits that accompany it. In addition, you won't experience any cravings, desire to binge, or strict dietary restrictions. If you have the patience to see the whole process through, instead of emotionally panicking at the first sign of weight gain and jumping on some five-hundred-calorie protein-shake diet—and if you go to great lengths to keep from compromising the items on the Metabolism Report Card along the way—you'll be handsomely rewarded. There are people who do practice this kind of thing. They are called "bodybuilders." No, you don't need to go to the same extremes as a bodybuilder, but the principles of human physiology apply to you, just as they do to someone on a psychotic quest to be as muscular and lean as is humanly possible.

If you are coming out of a diet state—whether you have been restricting fats, carbohydrates, or calories, or you've been creating a starvation state through excessive physical activity—the following is the sequence of events you will go through in terms of your body composition.

During the first stage of metabolic recovery, fat will initially accumulate at a much faster rate around the abdomen than in other areas of the body. Some think this is due to the body's desire to add fat around the internal organs to protect them from hypothermia. Whatever the reason for the change, be prepared for it, and don't freak out or jump ship before the next wave of changes.

So, at the start you'll gain weight quickly, then your weight gain will slow, and then it will stop altogether. You might gain weight for only two weeks or for several months—maybe fifteen pounds the first month, ten pounds the second, five pounds the third, and then finally none by the fourth month. I recommend just getting the weight-gaining part over with. Gaining fat is horrifying. When you stop gaining weight, it's quite a relief and you can focus more on completing your recovery. As I mentioned, I call the point of reaching zero fat gain while eating enormous quantities of even the most palatable and "fattening" food as becoming "fat-proof." Fat-proofing yourself is a very important first step.

It's also really important to take this process to completion. At first you gain weight around the abdomen, but then the rest of your body will fill out—adding more subcutaneous fat, which is generally believed to be highly protective and actually healthy. And, increasingly, your weight gains will consist of restored organ mass, bone mass, muscle mass, and glycogen storage. In other words, the *last* ten pounds you may gain during recovery are the most important pounds. Those pounds restore you to full capacity and also improve how your body looks. You can improve results even more by doing some progressive strength training during the process—not unlike the customary bodybuilding practice of going through a "bulk-up."

In other words, coming immediately out of a diet state you gain mostly fat and water. Let's say 90 percent of your weight gain is *not* lean tissue. After a few weeks, 50 percent of your weight gain might be healthy, lean tissue. After a couple of months you might be gaining 90 percent lean tissue, and eventually you will reach the point where weight gain stops completely. I've even communicated with people who continue to buy smaller and smaller pants as the numbers on their scales keep climbing.

Naturally, everyone wants to know how you can skip the fat gain and simply gain the lean mass. Sorry, the body just doesn't work that way. It's the gain in fat that raises the hormones that build lean tissue—youth-associated hormones, such as testosterone, progesterone, pregnenolone, and DHEA. You can't ever reach your highest health and aesthetic ideals without raising these hormones, and you can't raise those hormones without gaining at least a little body fat.

Once all that has taken place and your body is overflowing with healthy lean tissue and youthful hormones, much of the abdominal fat will start to redistribute itself throughout the rest of your body. At that point, you *may* start losing body fat spontaneously. If you don't, a reasonable increase in your physical activity levels is often enough to lose the extra fat without compromising the healthy tissue you've built.

Our biggest fear is that we will gain fat and never stop gaining or, if and when we do stop gaining, we won't be able to lose it. The body just doesn't work that way. It has many mechanisms to put the brakes on fat storage. For one thing, your metabolism will get high enough that stress hormones favoring fat storage (like cortisol) will bottom out. For another, after eating calorie-dense foods you desire until your appetite is fully satisfied and perhaps gaining a little fat, appetite falls precipitously. In fact, cravings and the compulsion to binge disappear completely, the desire and threshold for exercise typically soar, further fat gain becomes next to impossible without force-feeding yourself, and fat loss comes very easily.

This formula for metabolic recovery is basically the exact opposite set of changes that you experience when dieting and hitting a plateau. Instead of priming yourself for fat gain, you are priming yourself for effortless weight loss. It's really that simple. And best of all, you don't have to deprive yourself, go hungry, force yourself to do a lot of unwanted exercise, or do anything that resembles hard work and self-discipline. You also retain more muscle mass, making it possible to achieve a much more impressive fit and toned look than can be achieved through self-starvation.

Whether male or female, you will find that you eventually end up looking more muscular with more prominent fertile characteristics—a more masculine, muscular look for men, a more feminine hourglass figure and curvy look for women, with larger breasts and buttocks. The ultimate metric for aesthetic sex appeal is proportions.

Women, I can assure you that if your breasts and buttocks get larger in proportion to your waist, even if your waist gets a couple inches larger, you will look sexier—especially to males with high testosterone levels. Sex appeal is transmitted in much subtler ways as well: A rise in progesterone, regardless of your body fat levels, will make your face more attractive and even make your voice sound more feminine.

And men, the same is true for you. The more masculine you are, the more attractive you are (generally speaking) to women. A rise in metabolism, muscle mass, and testosterone does everything from subtly changing your face to giving you the iconic broad shoulders and full chest of your typical superhero. For some great lessons on sexual attraction, the documentary *The Science of Sex Appeal* is pretty interesting and accurate.

Metabolic rehab takes a solid year. Think of it as one step back, two steps forward. I think you'll be pleasantly surprised by the results, in both your health and the way you look.

Well, lookie there. I've droned on too long. No real surprise there. I hope I haven't scrambled your brain too much or made nutrition sound too complicated; it really isn't. The point is to experiment and pay careful attention to how your body responds.

The single biggest hindrance to good health and weight loss I've seen in health seekers is allowing way too much intellectual interference to stand between dietary choices and what are clear and obvious cries from the body for something completely different. Nutritional ideas that "make a lot of sense" or that you are 100 percent certain are correct are the most dangerous. The main takeaway is that good function comes first and nutritional philosophy comes second. Take that to heart and you're already way ahead of everyone else trying to eat their way to perfect health based on the latest popular trend.

PART

3

[E·X>E+R÷C=I×S-E]

Dr. Garrett Smith

Chapter 16
HEALTH VERSUS FITNESS

There is a necessity for a regulating discipline of exercise that, whilst evoking the human energies, will not suffer them to be wasted.

—Thomas de Quincey

A h, the exercise section. This is the part that is nearest and dearest to my heart. It was sports that originally led me to strength training, which led me to nutrition, which led me to medicine. What's the gist of this chapter? Don't Paleo fans already know that physical movement and exercise are of critical importance to health? Surely most of us do, and we have a basic familiarity with the long list of beneficial physiological changes that come with proper amounts and types of exercise.

I believe that most people who read this don't need a lecture on why physical movement is necessary and good for you, so I won't give you one. That said, I think many of us have found ourselves overanalyzing, overcompensating, and generally overdoing our physical activity in an elusive and impossible search for "optimal health." Often this runs completely parallel to what many of us do (or did) nutritionally. Too much info, too many rules, too many things to include or avoid—it all leads to paralysis by analysis and accompanying health issues (mainly from worrying too much about the perfect combination). Some of us have taken physical activity to extremes, even to the point of dependency and addiction.

If you're reading this chapter hoping to find some fitness holy grail—the last word on getting chiseled abs, achieving elite fitness (whatever that means), or getting "hyooge and swole" like the other bros—you're in the wrong place. Contrary to prevailing arguments, physical fitness *does not equal health*. My purpose and intent in this section is to provide you with concepts you can utilize to make exercise an almost wholly positive influence on your health, as well as to extend the years in which you can pursue the exercises of your choice.

First things first. Here are some of the exercise and movement concepts I live by.

1. The people who live the longest generally do lots and lots of low-intensity movement in the course of a day, with occasional (read: less often, not more often) higher-intensity systemic loads. Based on the research in *The Blue Zones* and on supercentenarians like Jeanne Calment (who, at 122 years, had the longest confirmed human life span in history), the exercises that facilitate longevity are enjoyable, consistent, sustainable, and natural. They are also done outside as much as possible—things like walking, gardening, hiking, and farming (including the raising and herding of animals). Real-world evidence proves that these provide long-term health benefits.

2. Movement is generally good. Inactivity (sitting) is bad. The more low-intensity movement you get per day, the better! Standing is better than sitting, walking is better than standing. Standing and walking during the day—for those with office jobs, think standing desks or walking treadmill desks—helps to increase your energy expenditure and metabolism without necessarily increasing your appetite (the way moderate- and high-intensity exercises do).

3. Exercise counts, period. Three ten-minute sessions of exercise is just as good as a single session of thirty minutes. If your job gives you the freedom to exercise in your office, you could split up your twenty sets of strength training exercises over a day, rather than jamming them all into an hour at the gym. Spreading your workout throughout the day is less stressful to your body than doing it all in one hour, and research shows that you will still get all the benefits.

4. The greatest reduction in mortality comes from the first twenty minutes of exercise.

5. Physical movement is totally necessary for proper brain development and maintenance.

6. After reaching a certain physical fitness standard, it can often be maintained by training once a week.

7. Exercise is a stress factor that we can control, for better or worse. Use this concept to your advantage. When life stressors are high in number and intensity, find and implement forms of stress-relieving exercise. Don't add to overall life stress by training hard at the wrong times.

8. Exercise should be fueled properly! Training while fasting or while consuming inadequate nutrition (low carbs, in particular) requires that your body create more blood sugar via gluconeogenesis. This is a fancy term that describes an increasing output of stress hormones (particularly adrenaline and cortisol) to enable self-cannibalization of your hard-earned muscle and some body fat. The higher intensity your workouts, the more carbs you require in your system to avoid this. Exercise is a stress, underfueling is a stress, high-intensity exercise is a massive stress. Two (or three) wrongs have never made a right. If you think you feel and perform better exercising on less food, do some Internet research on the "hunger high" and the "catecholamine honeymoon." I'll bet you'll reconsider.

Bottom line? The lion's share of major benefits to your health takes less exercise than you probably think. This is a critical point that contradicts just about everything you will read about fitness. In the next sections, I will encourage you to return to saner levels of activity.

Chapter 17

THE TROUBLE WITH TOO MUCH EXERCISE

Ninety percent of my time is spent holding athletes back to prevent overtraining, and only 10 percent is spent motivating them to do more work.

—Charlie Francis

First, a few basic facts. Is all exercise good? *No!* Can exercise be detrimental to health if done excessively? *Yes!* Do you have to move your body regularly in order to experience the greatest levels of health? *Absolutely!*

The reasons *why* you exercise are of extreme importance. In fact, you should have a mission statement for your workout program, and your decisions regarding exercise should always align with that mission. Sadly, that's not true for most people. For example, Matt and I have both worked with many people whose goals are low body-fat levels or "elite work capacity" because they have the misguided belief that these are synonymous with greater levels of health. Getting and staying healthy was their mission, but they were using the wrong markers to gauge their progress. If they were getting healthier, they wouldn't have been consulting with us, right? Refer back to Matt's list of metabolism indicators and use those as your markers for health. Really think about whether or not you are moving toward or away from those markers, and then reconsider your current exercise program.

Choices are always being made when it comes to exercise. Maybe you say your main reason for exercising is to improve your health. So, on a day when you have to choose between a healthy amount of sleep or cutting short your sleep so you can get in your workout, what choice do you make? The workout may help you improve your fitness at some cost to your overall health. This is reality, and it's another example of why fitness has never equaled health. So it's important to be honest with yourself about your goals. If you want to be the best in the world at something in your twenties—if you subject yourself to extreme diets to gain or lose weight, if you dehydrate yourself to "make weight," if you take performance-enhancing drugs—be aware that you have a real chance of significantly shortening your life through the choices you make. I'm not saying that you should deny yourself a dream, but do be aware of the consequences.

The current trend in exercise is "high-intensity" or "high-effort" training. A simple definition of these two terms means that you are working toward the upper ends of your capacity, whether in weight used, repetitions, heart rate, power output, distance, speed, or whatever other metric you use. All of this is hard to do and requires an unsustainable level of exertion. This is not a good thing for the average Joe or Jane who is simply interested in general physical fitness. Too much intensity or effort (read: stress)—whether in strength, endurance, or metabolic training—can cause irreparable damage to your hormonal systems.

Maybe you are fan of the "what doesn't kill you makes you stronger" fitspiration-type BS. If you are, I have four words for you: post-traumatic stress disorder (PTSD). It is important to know that the neuroendocrine profile (i.e., neurotransmitter and hormone levels) of overtraining is almost exactly the same as that of PTSD. Now, PTSD won't kill you, but it sure won't make you better (read: stronger) at dealing with stress! The body has a breaking point, as pioneering endocrinologist Dr. Hans Selye discovered a long time ago, and that breaking point can be reached gradually or within a single massively traumatic event.

What if you have overexercised? The first thing you need to know is that a week off from training won't solve your problem. Some of the damage you've suffered may be permanent. Think of joint or muscle injuries you may have had; sometimes the injury is small enough to heal well, but if the damage is never addressed or is continually aggravated, tissues may permanently change in a bad way. This is analogous to tendonitis (a simple inflammation of a tendon, often from overuse) versus tendinopathy (long-term negative tissue changes to a tendon from chronic tendonitis that has been continually reaggravated). Consider that the very same thing can happen to your nervous system and your endocrine system.

Ever heard a washed-up, broken athlete say, "I was never the same after [a particular program or event]"? He crossed the line of stress damage and never recovered. It's not just about getting older; it's that his chosen form of exercise and related stressors were actually aging him more quickly. Warning: The more mentally tough you are, the easier it is to damage yourself in this way because you find it easy to ignore or deny the warning signs.

As Hans and Franz would say,
"Hear me now, believe me later!"

Chapter 18
EXERCISE ADDICTION

I'm addicted to exercising and I have to do
something every day.

—Arnold Schwarzenegger

A sk yourself two very important series of questions:

1. Over the years, have you found it necessary to significantly increase the intensity or duration of your exercise in order to get the same physical and emotional benefits? If you don't feel drained or exhausted at the end of a workout session, do you find yourself complaining that "it wasn't hard enough"? Have one-hour workouts evolved into two hours, or even more?

2. If you don't get exercise on a regular basis—as in every day or every other day—do you experience any of the following emotional symptoms: anxiety, restlessness, irritability, insomnia, poor concentration, or depression? Or, put another way: Have people told you that when you don't work out, they notice that you become increasingly cranky, moody or unpleasant?

Sounds a little like addiction, doesn't it? I'll answer that for you. Yes, it does.

The questions above focus on the two main components of addiction—tolerance (needing more of something over time in order to get the same effect) and withdrawal (symptoms that appear when something habitually used or performed is taken away). Tolerance and withdrawal symptoms are markers of addiction, whether it's addiction to alcohol, cocaine, tobacco, or exercise.

Tolerance means that a person's reaction to a psychoactive compound (often this term refers to pharmaceutical or recreational drugs—we'll get to that in a second) decreases over time so that larger doses are required to achieve the same effect. Charlie Sheen may come to mind. If you find that you need two-plus hours of exercise a day to avoid withdrawal symptoms, or if you are pushing yourself harder and harder to get what you consider a decent workout, that is tolerance smacking you in the face.

If you're the type of person who doesn't feel "normal" if you miss a day or two of exercise, or if you get irritable when you don't exercise strenuously enough or long enough, you are also likely experiencing other symptoms of withdrawal, typically including anxiety, restlessness, insomnia, headaches, poor concentration, depression, and social isolation. If the exercise you're doing is truly good for you, your emotional state should not quickly deteriorate if you don't exercise for a couple of days.

Fitness addicts will say things like, "But exercise is good for me and I *need* it!" That's their way of justifying their high. Since lack of exercise is so common today, it must be a great thing that they are so dedicated to it, right? The reality for these folks is that exercise has simply become a method of self-medicating with stress hormones.

That being said, I also want to stress that *proper* exercise is the greatest antidepressant known to humankind, so I'm not surprised when people tell me they don't exercise and are depressed. It's the middle ground we're after: regular exercise that helps you feel good and improve your quality of life, without making you cranky and nasty if you miss a couple days.

I have personal experience with exercise addiction and many of the common fitness pursuits that are associated with it, including CrossFit, triathlon, powerlifting, kettlebells, and Olympic weight lifting. After recovering from all that, I researched the relationships among various endogenous psychotropic substances (our body's mood-controlling chemicals) that play major roles in exercise addiction. Keep in mind that these processes are involved in any kind of exercise, whether it's long-distance running (heard of the "runner's high"?) or the short-term, ammonia-snorting, face-slapping powerlifter's single repetitions. Boot campers, bodybuilders, and P90X-er types, don't worry: There's room for you, too.

First, the hook. Here's a common scenario. Many high-intensity-type gyms offer a free group workout to first-timers. These workouts are often *way* beyond the capacity of these people. They are designed that way! (I liken it to a drug dealer hooking potential customers with a free sample). Some newbies do the workout, feel awful, and never go back. But some do it and become instantly hooked on the stress hormone high, even as they lie in a pool of their own sweat (and possibly vomit) afterwards. Before long, they've sworn off all other forms of exercise and start disparaging those who don't go 100 percent 24/7. Been there, done that.

So what are they getting hooked on? Some people like to talk about preworkout, periworkout (during the workout), and postworkout nutrition. Instead of things people put in their body, let's discuss the natural substances triggered within the body before, during, and after high-intensity exercise. These substances operate much like drugs; they are present in the body all the time, but they drastically increase during different parts of a workout.

The preworkout "medication" for the exercise addict is the hormone adrenaline, or epinephrine, which triggers the body's fight-or-flight response—an extremely intense feeling sometimes called a "rush." Exercise addicts often talk about being nervous before particularly strenuous workouts. Here's a typical quote from a trainer deep in this mind-set: "If your workout doesn't scare you, it's not hard enough. If it scares you into staying home, then you're not hard enough." If something is scaring you, you've got your adrenaline switched on. But guess what? Fear and adrenaline are not positive things for health or metabolism. I'm sure you've heard the term "adrenaline junkies," which is the perfect way of describing people who get their high from self-inducing the fight-or-flight response through intentionally engaging in stressful or risky behavior.

Endorphins are the periworkout "medication." Maybe you think that a major benefit of exercise is the release of these chemicals, because they give people a pleasurable "endorphin rush," or "runner's high." Maybe . . . but maybe not. Let's break down the word *endorphin*: *endo* means "from within"; *orphin* means "morphine." Yes, endorphins are your body's very own version of morphine, a powerful opiate. Our own most common endorphin is one hundred times more powerful than morphine, which also likely means it is much more addictive. With sufficiently intense exercise, endorphins are released into the bloodstream and reach the brain. Sure, the runner's high is nice, but shouldn't it be a warning sign that the body feels the need to release powerful painkillers into the bloodstream? I would say it is! In all likelihood, there is enough tissue damage and pain occurring that the body decided it should self-medicate with a powerful opiate. In other words, the very thing that makes us feel happy during exercise is one of the things that cause addiction. The authors of a 2008 study titled "The Runner's High: Opioidergic Mechanisms in the Human Brain" wrote:

> In conclusion, this study provides the first in vivo evidence **that release of endogenous opioids occurs in frontolimbic brain regions after sustained physical exercise** and that there is its close correlation to perceived euphoria of runners. This suggests a specific role of the opioid system in the generation of the runner's high sensation. In a more general view, it might also be assumed that opioidergic effects in frontolimbic brain structures mediate not only some of the therapeutically beneficial consequences of endurance exercise on depression and anxiety in patients . . . but also the **addictive aspects of excessive sports, where injured athletes continue their training in spite of detrimental consequences to their health.** (emphasis mine)

If you have a chronically achy body part that hurts a bit when you start exercising and then feels better once you've "warmed it up" (your body just medicated itself with some endorphins, don't fool yourself), only to have the pain come back with a vengeance two hours after you've trained, that's my unscientific way of knowing that you are using endorphins as a painkiller. It's not that the joint got cold; it's that your drugs wore off!

Postexercise, who wouldn't want to relax? Here's where the body's endocannabinoid system (*endo* means, again, "from within," and cannabinoids are the various chemical constituents of cannabis, such as THC or cannabidiol) comes into play. Research has demonstrated that endocannabinoids are released in the brain during significantly intense exercise. The endocannabinoid system is involved in physiological processes like pain sensation (yes, it's another painkiller!), mood, appetite, and memory.

In short, we have a stimulant to get us hopped up before and during exercise, a painkiller to help us endure (and even enjoy) the damage we're doing to ourselves during exercise, and a sedative painkiller to help us relax afterwards. While these are not the only substances released by the body during intense physical activity, they are what I believe are the major players in exercise addiction. Seriously, who could resist getting highly attached to a free cocktail of adrenaline, morphine, and ganja? It makes me chuckle when I hear former drug addicts talking about how much better it is to be addicted to fitness than to smack. Little do they realize that they never kicked the drugs at all, they just found a new source.

Let's review the "perfect storm" for exercise addiction:

1. The chemicals our own bodies release during exercise are stronger than the street drug versions. These chemicals have very potent energy-producing, mood-enhancing, painkilling, and relaxing effects.

2. Getting "high" off exercise is not only legal but also encouraged by our culture.

3. Much like excessive water drinking, people tend to think that there is almost no such thing as too much exercise.

4. It is difficult for concerned friends and family to confront exercise addicts, because who wants to tell someone not to exercise?

Instead of wondering how people get addicted to exercise, I tend to wonder how people *don't* get addicted to exercise! Noticing the symptoms of withdrawal and tolerance are the first steps toward realizing an exercise addiction exists—feeling crappy if you don't get it, and always needing an increased "dose" in an impossible attempt to reach that initial high again. In the drug world, the latter is referred to as "chasing the dragon." Here's a tip-off: Nobody ever catches it.

It's time to get real. If you are experiencing signs of exercise addiction, the first step is admitting you have a problem, right? The next step is breaking the addiction cold turkey. Don't worry; we'll get to that.

Chapter 19
GENERAL GUIDELINES FOR SUSTAINABLE EXERCISE

To me, the sign of a really excellent routine is one that places great demands on the athlete, yet produces progressive long-term improvement without soreness, injury, or the athlete ever feeling thoroughly depleted. Any fool can create a program that is so demanding that it would virtually kill the toughest marine or hardiest of elite athletes, but not any fool can create a tough program that produces progress without unnecessary pain.

—Dr. Mel C. Siff

Do as little as needed, not as much as possible.

—Henk Kraaijenhof

Stimulate, don't annihilate.

—Lee Haney

This chapter contains general guidelines for a workout program that facilitates sustainability, consistency, and long-term progress. None of the points are new, nor are they uniquely mine. They have worked for my patients and me again and again. If you want to keep moving and exercising for the rest of your life (and I hope you do), the following training guidelines will serve you well.

Once again, if your goal is to be a so-called elite athlete, disregard the following mantra: You have made a choice to sacrifice your health in exchange for fitness. Keep in mind that great health and extreme training do not go together, but if you want to pursue an extreme training regimen, then go for it. However, if your goal is to be physically capable, with exercise and movement adding both quality and years to your life, then study the following carefully.

Here we go.

[1]
Take some time off. Break the habit

Let's say you saw yourself in the exercise addiction section—as in, you realized that your face should be next to the definition of *exercise addiction* on Wikipedia. You've now decided that you want to regain control of your life. You don't do it by tapering off. That's similar to the bad advice some people give alcoholics: If you want to stop the problem, just reduce the amount you're drinking. Is that a good plan? "No" would be the correct response.

For addicts, simply reducing use has never been—nor will it ever be—a good solution. So let's adopt a lesson from the rehab world: Go cold turkey. Attempts at weaning will *absolutely fail* if you're in charge of your own training. In my experience, three days of abstaining from exercise will break the main physiological and biochemical addiction to exercise, but it takes three weeks to break the habit entirely.

The fastest way to break an exercise addiction and reap the benefits is to take four to six weeks off—*completely off!* Just in case you're still unclear: That means *no exercise!* Some people need this spelled out a bit more. No counting reps or sets. No fitness classes of any type. No competitive games or sports. No heart rate monitors or any other measuring devices. There is a method to this. You will not die if you don't train for six weeks, nor will you actually lose much strength at all. If you find your skin crawling after two to three days, that's the withdrawal talking; it means you need to press on. That part will go away, I promise.

What if you simply must do *something*? Take a stroll—and by *stroll* I mean a "slow walk." I don't mean a power walk or a slow jog or a hike up a mountain. You may also do some easy stretching or take a super-easy yoga class (hot yoga is out). If you have a physically demanding job, do your work, taking it as easy as possible, and skip any other exercise. If you bike to work, consider taking the bus or driving instead for this period.

If you fall into the "overexercise-addict" category, you've probably dug yourself into a hole that you were unaware you were even digging. Maybe you're still not sure if it's a hole that you want or need to get out of. Or maybe you (or your dumb trainer or coach) think training even harder is the way out. You might even be prodding your tired body onward each day by posting "fitspiration" memes—trite motivational sayings combined with pictures of super-fit people—on social networking sites to keep yourself motivated while disregarding the obvious signs your body is giving you. How have these things worked out for you so far? Not so well? It could be that many things you thought were right are completely wrong.

There is only one way to get out of the exercise addiction cycle. Commit 100 percent to no exercise for four to six weeks. If you aren't sure if it is "exercise" or not, don't do it. Also realize that, just like any other addiction, you may struggle the rest of your life trying to balance the human body's need for exercise without falling back into exercise-addiction patterns.

When your body begins to recover, you may find you have gained a natural aversion to the types and amounts of exercise that you had been subjecting your body to for so long; in the future you will be better able to determine what is good for you and what is damaging. The benefits of this for your general health will be incredible. You are not a wuss for not wanting to do overly intense exercise any longer.

Conversely, and particularly at the early stages, you may find yourself lapsing back into the more/harder/heavier exercise pattern of an addict. Notice it and shut it down sooner rather than later. Personally, I find that training by myself makes it easiest to resist those urges. Group training and classes tend to feed exercise addiction.

[2]
Recognize the activities that stimulate a fight-or-flight response

This is going to sound obvious, but fighting, sparring, rolling, and other types of martial arts or confrontational activities will fire up your stress hormones. (Duh! See the word *fight* in *fight-or-flight*.) You have one stress button, and everything stressful pushes it. Being in physical danger is one of the most acutely stressful things that can happen to you, whether you choose to admit it or not.

If you have a job that constantly stimulates your fight-or-flight response (for instance, you're in the police or fire department or the military), you will have to work very hard to balance your stressful work activities with stress-relief practices. (See Part Four: Sleep and Recovery for ideas.)

[3]
Do not train extra hard to "burn off stress"

Say you're in a stressed state because of (pick one or more) work, kids, school, money, fasting, whatever. Cool (not really, actually it sucks, but *c'est la vie*). It happens to everyone at some point. What are you going to do about it?

"Grrrrr! Today sucked. I'm gonna go crush myself with [fill in your choice of excessively intense exercise here] and work it off!"

On a particularly stressful day, your stress button has already been pushed many times. Maybe it's left you feeling achy, tired, and anxious. Now you're going to go push the button again by beating yourself up with the stress of intense exercise? If you read the last chapter, on exercise addiction, you now know why you want to exercise hard: to get that endorphin (aka super-morphine) plus adrenaline (epinephrine) plus endocannabinoid (aka marijuana-related) fix! Sure, it feels good for an hour or two, but underneath that brief euphoria is a whole lot of stress damage you'll have to deal with later.

Training too hard on stressful days is a double whammy in the wrong direction. (Matt's not the only guy who can use the term *double whammy!*) Be smarter; don't do it. On bad days, regardless of what you might have planned, do something that truly relieves stress, not something that creates more of it. Stick with recovery types of workouts, like easy cardio, a nice walk outside, or some painless stretching or mobility work.

[4]
Listen to your body

Everybody has gut feelings. Most people don't pay attention to them, and that's part of the reason Matt and I wrote this book. If your gut is telling you that today is not a good day to train or exercise, take the hint. The first sign your body gives off in a stressed state is an aversion to further stressors! Don't force yourself to push through the lack of motivation or the pain or the exhaustion. Take a day off.

That said, my personal rule before taking a day off training is to at least do my warm-up. If I do my warm-up and perk up, then I will continue with the workout. If I do my warm-up and still feel like I want to go home, then I take the hint and go home. For most of us, our daily jobs are not physically exhausting, but they are mentally exhausting. A good warm-up will get oxygenated blood flowing through the brain and body, and you will often see the mental and physical fatigue disappear.

[5]
Spread your workout over your day

Research continually shows that we get the same benefits from exercise whether it is done in one large chunk or broken into multiple smaller chunks. This goes back to what I was saying in Chapter 16 about world's longest-lived groups—they are generally moving and doing physical things through most of their day. To me, it makes sense that spreading eight sets of an exercise throughout the day puts less stress on the system than doing the same eight sets in thirty minutes.

I realize that this isn't possible for everyone, but the concept is important. Spreading out the effort spreads out the stress. If you work in an office environment, your best options for this include walking (treadmill desk, anyone?), stairs, and body-weight exercises, aka calisthenics.

[6]
If you feel worse two hours after you finish your workout, then you did too much

This guideline is particularly important for those recovering from a significant history of overexercising and those dealing with health issues related to conditions such as reactive hypoglycemia, adrenal fatigue, and hypothyroidism.

The type of workout you've done doesn't matter. If you feel significantly worse—exhausted, in more pain, or overly emotional—two hours after a workout than you did before it, back off and do less next time. Listen to your body. If you follow this approach from the beginning of your recovery, you will be able to progress later. If you screw things up in the beginning, you'll remain stuck. By choosing to take a step backwards, you can eventually take two steps forward.

What's happening when you feel like a champ immediately after a workout, then feel like hell two hours later? Simple: You were fueling your workout with stress hormones and you came to the end of your exercise high.

This guideline is particularly important if you have aches or pains that feel better during a workout and then return or even intensify two hours later. Stress hormones numbed the pain, and when their effect wears off, you get to feel the damage that was done.

If you are exercising for your health and longevity, you should feel *better* (invigorated, even!) long after a workout. You should *not* feel worse. If you are always exhausted and sore—except when you're training hard—then you are sacrificing your current quality of life and likely your future health.

[7]
Pay attention to the quality of air you're breathing during exercise

I'm going to guess that if you're reading this book you're not a smoker and you think inhaling combustion by-products is generally a bad idea. So why would you exercise next to cars burning up fuel and giving you the automotive equivalent of secondhand smoke? Inhaling car and truck exhaust has been directly shown to lower testosterone and damage sperm.

Next, ever heard of sick building syndrome (SBS)? This means that the air inside a building may be of significantly worse quality than outside air. It happens quite often. Let me give you the air profile of an actual gym I've visited:

+ Located right on one of the city's busiest streets (where exhaust fumes are heavy)

+ Shares a wall and open drainage system with an auto transmission repair shop, so various solvent fumes and other volatile organic chemicals (VOCs) in the air are undoubtedly high

+ Smells from the rubber floor mats and bumper plates are off-gassing

+ Uses evaporative "swamp" cooling much of the year; this tends to promote the growth of mold

Your lungs are designed to absorb stuff from the air, for better or worse. Exercise that greatly increases your breathing rate will also increase your exposure to any unhealthy things in the air and may negatively impact your health over time. Pick a place and time to exercise where the air is clean(er). The simplest steps to take are to try to exercise outdoors, away from major roads, and not during rush-hour traffic.

Among the key indicators that you may be breathing nasty stuff during your workouts—assuming you don't have asthma or other respiratory issues already: During and/or after your workouts you get a nagging cough or a tightness or burning in your chest or throat. Pay attention. Good exercise plus bad air will likely exacerbate health problems.

[8]
Do not do "constantly varied" or "pseudorandom" or "muscle confusion" programs

There are three good reasons to stick with the same exercises in your program for significant periods, instead of constantly changing things (a fairly recent exercise fad).

A. Habituation

The body gets used to stimuli (like squats) through repetition. This means that over time and with repetition, your body will release fewer stress hormones for the same amount of work. This is a good thing. If you've ever heard of the SAID principle (Specific Adaptation to Imposed Demands) or the concept of "If you want to get better at doing X, then you need to practice X regularly," that's what we're talking about. Through practice and repetition, you get better at what you do, and in most cases *better* means you're doing it with less stress and greater efficiency. The reduced stress hormone release after repetition has been documented in activities as stressful as parachuting; squats are nothing in comparison to that!

Frequent introduction (and reintroduction) of new exercises, rep schemes, and entire workouts add variables that increase the amount of stress in the body. This is a bad thing over the long term. Try to stick with a set program for at least eight weeks before changing things.

B. Adaptation and preparation

Constantly changing your exercises means that your ability to gauge how much they impact you (both during and after your workout) is highly compromised. For example, if John Doe squatted 225 pounds for ten reps last week, he would know exactly how that made him feel. If he were to squat 235 pounds the next week, he'd have a good idea, before even starting, how many reps he'd likely accomplish and how much it would affect his recovery.

But let's say John Doe's brother got on the "muscle confusion" train. He squatted 225 pounds for ten reps last week, this week he wants to front squat, next week he wants to do lunges, and the week after that he wants to overhead-squat. To gain the most benefit, all these exercises will use different amounts of weight and probably need different numbers of repetitions. If he only repeats an exercise once a month, he can't really know how that exercise will affect him, which then affects his ability to plan for sessions to come in the near future. Failing to plan equals planning to fail. Constant soreness is a hallmark of programs that do not repeat themselves frequently enough to induce adaptation. Soreness should not be a goal of exercise. Chronic soreness is chronic inflammation, and that is a terrible thing for health.

C. Strength building

An exercise must be repeated often enough, with proper increases in resistance over time, for the body to get stronger. Pseudorandom training will not typically get one past novice levels of strength.

In summary, rotating exercises and rep schemes from day to day and week to week does not allow you to estimate ahead of time what you're in for, your stress systems will not adapt over time, and you will be limited to novice (maybe intermediate, if you are lucky) levels of strength. It's just a bad idea.

[9]
Limit hard conditioning sessions to a maximum of ten minutes per session, but closer to five is best

As competitive weight lifter Jim Wendler has said:

Most of my conditioning is done without much intensity; I relax and just get a quality workout in and leave. Do this consistently enough, however, and your conditioning goes through the roof. . . . I simply strive for good workouts done consistently. You'll be surprised at what happens when this is done, and it doesn't take long to realize the benefits.

Metabolic conditioning (met-con). Finishers. High-intensity circuit training (HICT). These are all general terms for a bunch of exercises done as quickly as possible. It's well-known for inducing rapid fat loss in the early phases, creating exercise addicts over time, and ending in burnout.

In my experience, these types of sessions are, hands down, the easiest way to overdo exercise. It's very difficult to quantify *effort* during this kind of conditioning. This is bad, mmkay?

For those of you drinking the met-con Kool-Aid and thinking I have no idea what I'm talking about, listen up. This was a major modification I made in Josh Everett's workouts in the time between his two podium finishes at the CrossFit Games.

My rule for doing strictly conditioning workouts, either on their own or after strength training, is that there is a strict limit on the amount of work time (five minutes preferably, ten at the most). Once that timer beeps, you are *done*. You don't finish a round just because you were "so close."

If you're that attached to your scores, you still aren't getting what I'm telling you. If you've ever heard that "men will die for points," I'm here to tell you that injuries and damage to your hormonal systems will come well before death, and they will make your life suck. Maybe you've already noticed.

Another important part of my rule for conditioning sessions is that whatever you choose to do needs to be "doable enough" (or *scaled,* if you prefer that term) that you're able to continually move the *entire time.* You should not have to stop to catch your breath, psych yourself up, get angry, or wait for your strength to return in order to do more reps.

Think of this as the conditioning version of avoiding training to muscular failure. Get stronger using strength training; get more conditioned through conditioning. Let that sink in a bit. Don't try to use one to build the other, and don't practice failing (unless you are trying to become better at failing). If you're interested in knowing more about this approach to conditioning, I've included several links in the references section.

If you feel worn down from previous excessive exercise or are a recovered exercise addict, I'm a big fan of leaving conditioning out of your regimen entirely. Once you reintroduce it, realize that a little bit of conditioning goes a long way. Improving your strength also improves your conditioning, but not so much the other way around.

[10]
Limit total cardio and long slow distance (LSD) training to a max of thirty minutes per session

Count your conditioning as time spent doing cardio training, if you are doing any. This means that over the course a day, I suggest you limit yourself to either thirty minutes of cardio or five minutes *max* of conditioning plus twenty-five minutes of cardio. Cardio training should stay in the aerobic zone, which is found by subtracting your age from 180. An example: I am thirty-seven years old, so my max cardio heart rate is 180 minus 37, or 143 beats per minute (credit to Phil Maffetone for that equation). I'll bet you'll find that these low-intensity cardio sessions will help you recover from other workouts better.

Long, moderate-to-high intensity cardio workouts are a surefire way to tire out your adrenals, toast your thyroid, and kill your metabolism. Do yourself a favor and stop doing them now!

[11]

Beware of any workout regimen that celebrates complete exhaustion, vomiting, or sending people to the hospital with rhabdomyolysis

Some of you will immediately recognize where this comes from. Some of you who know my background also know that I have significant experience with a regimen of this nature. I'll cover each one, but the main thing to realize is that programs that enable or encourage exhaustion, puking, and "rhabdo" are not healthy or sustainable.

A. Exhaustion

If you work out to exhaustion, you have thoroughly pushed the stress button many, many times. Now you're exhausted and you'll have to deal with the short- and long-term repercussions of what your self-induced stress hormone marinade does to your body. More critically, you will have made withdrawals from your stress savings account that can never be paid back. What if you eagerly go back for more? Well, you're probably an exercise addict.

If you're a follower of the Paleo ideals in our modern world, get this. Our Paleolithic ancestors would never have voluntarily exercised or exerted themselves to complete exhaustion unless their lives depended on it. Excessive voluntary exercise leads to two things that are bad for survival: exhaustion and increased food needs. A sore, exhausted caveman is a sitting duck for just about any dangerous situation!

B. Vomiting

If you're one of those people who thinks vomiting is the sign of a good workout or good effort, I'm sorry to burst your bubble. It's not a positive sign of anything other than pushing way too hard.

Here's what happened. Your blood sugar levels dropped extremely quickly at some point (common causes of this during exercise include low-carbing, fasted exercise, calorie-restrictive diets, and excessively long and/or intense training sessions). To avoid allowing your blood sugar to drop too low, your body dumped massive amounts of stress hormones into your system in order to turn fat and protein into more sugar (to keep you standing upright and conscious). This involves a desperate diversion of blood from your digestive system to your arms and legs. The result of all this? Say hello to your lunch for a second time. On a related note, dry heaving simply means you had nothing to send back up, but the same process happened anyway.

If your trainer pushes you to the point of puking on a regular basis and you continue to pay him or her, I don't know who is dumber. If your gym gives rewards like stickers or T-shirts for reaching this point, I suggest you find another place to exercise.

C. Rhabdomyolysis

The crowning achievement of exercise dumbassery is rhabdomyolysis, potentially a life-threatening condition!

It's defined as follows:

A condition in which skeletal muscle is broken down, releasing muscle enzymes and electrolytes from inside the muscle cells. Risks of rhabdomyolysis include muscle breakdown and kidney failure because the cellular component myoglobin is toxic to the kidneys. Rhabdomyolysis is relatively uncommon, but it most often occurs as the result of extensive muscle damage as, for example, in crush injury or electrical shock. Drugs or toxins may also cause this disorder. Underlying diseases that can also lead to rhabdomyolysis include collagen vascular diseases, such as systemic lupus erythematosus.

Is that serious enough for you? What is the point at which exercise crosses from healthy to unhealthy to possibly deadly? Do you want to try to find out? Understand that exercising to improve one's health should go in the exact opposite direction of creating this condition. Health and hospital visits? They don't go together.

It's beyond me how the idea of workouts resulting in multiday hospital stays that include IV fluids and pain medications (mainly morphine, ahem, an opiate)—or even death!—became equated with health.

Back in my days of training like an idiot, I probably reached a point of *very mild* rhabdomyolysis twice, based on my symptoms afterwards: abnormal amounts of pain and swelling in the affected regions, as well as tan-colored urine—not the cola-colored urine of more serious cases. One time it happened after overdoing glute-ham developer (GHD) sit-ups; the other time it was from pull-ups. I was lucky (smart?) enough to stop before I needed a hospital visit. However, for months after both events I had to roll to the side and push myself up to get off the ground (I couldn't "sit up" anymore), and I totally lost my ability to do pull-ups for a long while.

Does injuring your muscles and their nerve connections to the point where you are unable to do certain exercises *for several months* conjure up cool, tough-guy images in your brain, or does it sound like the stupidest thing you could possibly do? Please say the latter. Be smarter than this. If someone told you he had a habit that induced utter exhaustion, vomiting, and/or life-threatening muscle and kidney damage, you'd probably look at him in horror and tell him to stop that garbage, right? Exercise is no exception!

In the next section, I'll go over some of the training rules that I've found to be most effective in maximizing a workout's health-building components.

An Outdoor Life

Matt Stone

I grew up in Nashville, Tennessee. There, I found the concept of exercising to primarily mean "working out" or "training." I had that whole skateboarding phase that I went through. I played a lot of Wiffle ball and rode bikes all over my neighborhood. Beat the hell out of lightning bugs with a tennis racket. Caught more crawdads down at the creek than you can shake a stick at. But after about the sixth grade, exercise and even sports became divorced from play. Sure, those first twelve years of my life were incredibly fun, but at some point we have to get serious about all this exercise, right?

Twice during my developmental years I had the luxury of moving away from Tennessee and out to Colorado. My dad had a serious mountain man fetish, and so did I. (I watched *The Adventures of the Wilderness Family* about a thousand times growing up.) When I was nine, Pops had a little extra dough and decided to build a house in the absolute middle of nowhere. So we moved out to our glorified Kaczynski cabin several miles from our nearest neighbor and a thirty-five-minute drive to even the closest, tiny grocery store. We lived there for a whole year.

During that year I spent most of my time in the outdoors. I would hike all over our property, shooting at stuff with my little shotgun. Our closest neighbor had a small pond filled with way too many trout, and I walked a mile down there to fish almost every day. How could I not? The smallest trout in there was big by any standards and ten hogs would fight for my fly on every cast. I've been spoiled ever since!

Every Saturday in the winter, my parents threw me on a school bus full of kids dressed head to toe in ridiculous neon clothing. Saturday was ski school. For $10 every local kid could hitch a ride, ski all day, get some tasty food product for lunch, and get a ride back to town. That's just what kids did on Saturday. And often I would ski with my parents or some friends on Sunday. That's about twelve hours outdoors, having fun, and, incidentally, getting some tremendous exercise every weekend.

When we moved back to Nashville, I quickly noticed a trend. My friends never did anything outdoors. By the seventh grade, we were staying up all night playing video games. By ninth grade, socializing was pretty much drinking alcohol. Neat.

Thankfully, when I was sixteen, we moved back to Colorado. Back to hiking, fly-fishing, and skiing every weekend with friends (at sixteen, kids still did this all weekend, every weekend, all winter long, just as they did in the fourth grade), and even backpacking. Loading up with forty pounds of stuff and hiking miles up mountains was a far cry from standing around a keg with a plastic cup or playing video games until the sun came up. That wasn't the *only* thing we did in Nashville, but it certainly seemed like it.

Needless to say, I haven't spent much time in Nashville since. Instead, I have tended to gravitate to many of the world's outdoor recreation meccas. Sure, I got a little carried away, as you've read about already—turning this outdoor recreation stuff into some kind of forty-four-day Tough Mudder instead of letting it just be a fun and uplifting way to spend the time. But that's my own damn fault, certainly not the fault of the world that exists on the other side of the drywall.

The problem with exercise isn't necessarily what type you are doing; it's the whole concept of exercise itself. I live in Florida now and I lift some weights and work out some days, but I never forget to get outside merely for the sake of being outdoors. When I do fail to make it outside, it's not because I've forgotten how good it is for me. It's just that the indoor environment has many qualities that make it difficult to feel good and energetic and upbeat and happy enough to want to go outside and play! The indoor world is like the eternally gloomy, cloudy day that goes on forever.

For someone who has spent as much time as I have outdoors, I feel that I have a pretty unique perspective on it. I have done it enough to feel the physical changes it causes; the psychological quieting; the feeling of being fully in tune with the daily sunlight rhythms; the subtle contrast between fresh, flowing stream water and what comes out of the tap; the rejuvenation of sleeping on the ground for many weeks at a time. Being outside is different. We can speculate as to why that is, and Garrett will soon discuss several scientifically valid reasons behind it, but being outdoors, recreating freely, without attaching any concepts of intervals or plyometrics or training to it, is one of the most health-enhancing experiences I can think of.

Perhaps the reason I am most compelled to encourage you to give priority to outdoor recreation over traditional exercise in all its many forms is that I've seen the real-life, observable, cumulative benefits of it. The fitness, agility, athleticism, and all-around terrific physiques of the people living in areas where outdoor recreation is a way of life are abundantly clear, especially as these people enter their fifties, sixties, and beyond. It's not like there's a big obesity epidemic in Aspen, Colorado, or Jackson Hole, Wyoming—two of the many places I have lived. They eat plenty of pizza and drink ample amounts of beer in these places, too, I assure you! And gyms? In these places they are scarce and usually completely empty except for the climbing wall, which occupies most of the gym space.

No treadmill or exercise program could ever compete with getting ten, twenty, or even more hours of fun and enjoyable outdoor exercise per week. Plus, who could force themselves to work out in a gym for as long as they can when they are simply having fun? So make getting outside your number-one priority—for no reason other than it's better to be out *doing* something than it is to be sitting around inside. It just so happens you will feel better physically; have greater mobility, flexibility, and fitness; and be a heck of a lot more energetic and happy if you stop working out so hard, stop sitting around waiting for Facebook to complete you in some way, and start having more fun.

If you need verifiable 'scientifically based' reasons to do it (dear Lord, I hope you don't), Garrett has some in store for you. But you shouldn't need a reason to drag yourself away from the stifling indoor prison that has become our modern way of life and out onto a surfboard, a pair of skis or snowshoes, the golf course, the local trail, your bike, or the pool. Even sitting outside on my porch to do all my computer work has made a tangible difference in my health and mood. I don't care how you get out there, but if you do you are unlikely to regret it—especially if you can leave the warrior mind-set and even the health mind-set in the house and the gym.

Play out more, work out less. There's simply no substitute for sunlight and fun outdoor recreation—and lots of it—not just for health enhancement but for life enhancement. And dude, it's like, so Paleo.

Chapter 20

YOUR NEW TRAINING RULES

My general rules for training are the same for everyone, whether you're a former exercise addict with a damaged metabolism, looking for a saner way to exercise, or just a normal person who wants to move and exercise in a healthy way for the rest of your life.

Most of these rules will fall into the "autoregulate" category, which in fancy terms means "a biological system equipped with inhibitory feedback systems such that a given change tends to be largely or completely counteracted."

What does this mean to you ("the biological system")? It means that I'm going to tell you the body's signals to watch for that indicate you should back off or stop. This will allow you to do your exercise in the proper amount and avoid traveling into the land of excessive stress. As long as you are aware of these signals, pay attention when they happen, and adjust what you are doing accordingly, you'll find them easy to incorporate into your training.

Strength Without Strain

Matt Stone

We live in a society that generally believes that working harder and pushing yourself to the highest level of strain possible will yield the greatest results. In some cases and in some circumstances, this might be true. But, ultimately, with exercise aimed at gaining strength or muscle or overall fitness, harder doesn't mean better. It certainly isn't better if your health is compromised in any way. We are not all elite athletes and freaks of nature. We have to work with what we've got, not against it.

Like most guys my age (thirty-five), I've done a great deal of huffing and puffing and grunting to the point where I'm dizzy and nauseous in the gym—and I never got exceptional long-term results. I don't possess the threshold of elite athletes. I definitely don't have the threshold of people who are both genetically blessed *and* taking a bunch of illicit drugs to further increase their threshold for self-punishment. Even if the most grueling of all conceivable routines were the key for those who become world-champion bodybuilders, strength athletes, or fitness athletes, that doesn't mean *you* won't end up sick and hurt or just totally burned out if you try to place the same demands on your body.

In reality, if we're talking strictly in terms of increasing strength—probably the best barometer of structured exercise—odds are that your best results will come from a moderate—as in sustainable—approach.

By *moderate* and *sustainable* I mean "easy, quick, and safe"—as in not injuring yourself—while you make slow and steady progress. How hard do you have to push yourself to gain strength from week to week for many months and even years on end? Do you have to strain to squeeze in that one last, brutal rep? Do you have to be in the gym five days a week for an hour each round? Hell, no! In fact, if you do, you'll likely get some great gains for three months, but then you'll burn out or injure yourself, and then you'll be right back where you started (or even weaker) six months later when you get all gung-ho for another round of butt-kicking (only to repeat the same thing again, of course).

The net result is wear, tear, no progress, an increasingly negative relationship with exercise, and a defeatist attitude—with occasional bursts of irrational positivity (the gung-ho part of the cycle).

The good news is that there are numerous systems that lead to increased strength, and all of them require very little time and overall effort, including Jim Wendler's 5/3/1, Pete Cisco's Static Contraction or Power Factor Training methods, John Little and Doug McGuff's Body by Science, Bryan Haycock's Hypertrophy-Specific Training (HST), and a long list of others. You just have to keep adding weight, little by little, and when you can't add more weight, start taking more time off—not working harder and longer.

I've found that the less I do, the stronger I get. That's what a lot of the proponents of various "quick and easy" systems have discovered as well. More importantly, the less I do, the longer I stick with it. I don't think I've ever even seen the guy with the best physique at my gym break a sweat. But you know what? I come and go, and he's always coming in regularly, doing his easy-ass workout and making slow but steady and sustainable progress.

Ultimately, what works the best isn't what gives you the biggest muscles or the fastest weight loss. What works the best is what you'll still be doing many years from now.

I encourage you to think of training in a new way. Doug McGuff introduced me to the concept of the "minimum effective dose" when it comes to formal workouts. If you can get progressively stronger by lifting weights for fifteen minutes once every ten days, why go three times a week for an hour each time? The older you are, the more you have brutalized your body, and the more total stress burden your body and mind is under at any given time, the more important this becomes.

Be efficient. Get the most strength with the least amount of strain. You'll be surprised when you find out just how much you've been doing beyond what is necessary to get results. You'll also be surprised how much better you feel when you aren't in a perpetually bruised and battered state of recuperation.

Keep in mind, these tips are for health seekers, not elite or wannabe-elite athletes. Remember, to be a top-level athlete, you must consistently make choices supporting improved performance rather than improved health. The list of professional athletes who have reached one hundred years of age is amazingly short. You could take that fact as a cautionary tale.

[1]

No preworkout stimulants.

Thermogenics, "fat-burners," preworkout methylxanthines, ephedrine, nicotine, and synephrine are all stimulants and increase stress hormone levels by pharmaceutical means. The bodybuilding supplement industry seems to come out with new variants every week, each one with less human research done on it than the one before. The general effect of these products is to boost short-term energy levels at the expense of possible long-term health issues, particularly related to blood sugar control.

Maybe your reaction to this is, "I'm *so* tired. I need to exercise. If I don't have my herbal speed in a pill, my workout will suck. I *need* it to get through my workout!" My thoughts upon hearing something like that are similar to my thoughts about dependency and metabolic damage. Your exercise should be what's invigorating you, not pills or potions!

For special events or competitions, I'm not against using one of the greatest performance enhancers known to humankind: caffeine in coffee. Otherwise, tread carefully. Taking something every day or for every workout isn't moderation. It's a habit.

[2]

No psyching up for anything unless in competition.

Why? "Psyching up" is about inducing the release of stress hormones into your system for the purpose of doing more (reps, weight, whatever). This includes requiring music to amp yourself up, heavy and fast breathing, growling, yelling, or just generally inducing anger and hyperarousal before you start a set.

If you've been training for years, you may have noticed that the psyching-up process for heavy sets gets more difficult over time, your prelift routines get longer and more intense, and it all just seems to suck more life out of you afterwards. If you're at the point where lifting more requires sniffing ammonia or someone slapping you, you're a long way down this road! When you rely on your stress hormones too often, your body adapts and requires more stimuli over time. For those addicted to heavy lifting, this is one place where tolerance rears its ugly head.

Save the psyching up for fitness testing or actual competitions— both defined here as an event where you truly give 100 percent effort, whether you are competing for awards or trophies or not. I would suggest a maximum of six competitions per year, and limiting yourself to three is probably better.

Psyching up is probably the most stressful and draining thing people do in their training. Set your ego aside, stop doing it, and your health will benefit greatly.

[3]
"No face strain" (NFS) during slow or grinding lifts, and stop your set when rep speed noticeably slows down.

This is the hardest rule for most people to stick with, yet it's the most beneficial in the long term. On the slow or grinding lifts (squats, presses, dead lifts, machines, etc.), don't make a face while doing sets or reps, regardless of how many you do. If you start to scrunch your cheek, squint your eyes, clench your teeth, purse your lips, whatever, your set is *done.*

Face strain means that your body is becoming stressed and is digging deeper into its reserve systems to create more tension in order to complete the job. Think of your face as an indicator of how much your body is being stressed, because, really, how much weight are your face muscles lifting?

By not allowing this to happen—or not allowing it to progress past the initial point of noticing it—you can continue to lift decent weight without cutting into your recovery. This may initially require a reduction of 30–50 percent in your work set weights; you'll have to figure this out for yourself. I have seen people training in this method eventually lift 90 percent of their one-rep max weights for single reps with NFS.

Maybe you think improvement is impossible without face strain. I disagree. Watch male Olympic gymnasts in competition. Unless they are in the middle of a ballistic move, their faces are without noticeable strain or emotion—and they stay that way. If some of the world's strongest and most coordinated athletes can avoid face strain while doing some of the hardest moves around *during competition,* do you really think you need to make faces in your local gym?

The second part of this rule is about rep speed. At some point in a set, there is generally a point where you will notice an obvious slowing of rep speed. Cut the set off there; this is where form starts going in the toilet, so take the hint. Maintaining proper form nearly all the time (no "20 percent slop" acceptable here) is a hallmark of those who train successfully over *decades.*

So here's how a single set would look: no psych-up to start, NFS through the set, and the set ends when any of the following has happened:

+ **You reach your target number of reps with NFS.**

+ **You break NFS and stop the set after that rep, regardless of whether you hit any arbitrary rep goal or not.**

+ **You notice your rep speed significantly and obviously slowing down. Stop the set after that rep. Again, this is regardless of whether you hit your rep goal or not.**

As I stated above, you will need to begin this new approach by checking your ego at the door and lowering your weights. With time and practice, you'll be able to handle higher percentages of your actual one-rep max with NFS. You won't accomplish this if you don't back way off at the beginning; some people have to go down to approximately 50 percent of their one-rep max before they can unlearn the nasty face-strain habit. (You might need to have someone spot you at first, to let you know when it is happening, as exercise addicts are masters of denial and self-delusion. I know. I used to be one and I still have occasional lapses.) Have a slice of humble pie and do yourself a long-term favor.

NFS does not apply to explosive movements like Olympic weight lifting, kettlebell ballistic lifts, or plyometrics; this technique doesn't work well for them (except maybe kettlebell swings). Regarding explosive or ballistic weight training, as I get older, I'm finding more and more truth to this quote from *The Lifting Cure* by David P. Butler, originally published in 1868:

> With slow movements, though the weights are heavy, one is always prepared to restrain action short of rupture or strain; while, in quick movements, the action is beyond the control of the person. He knows liability only when he is injured.

The truth in Butler's quote is clear in the participation rates of Masters-age athletes in powerlifting and Olympic weight lifting, respectively. The slower lifts of powerlifting (squat, bench press, dead lift) have a much higher percentage of Masters participants than the ballistic snatch and clean-and-jerk lifts of Olympic weight lifting. How you use this information is up to you.

[4]
No failure at any point during a workout.

As competitive powerlifter Dave Tate has said:

> If you just want to look good for the beach and be stronger than the average guy there's absolutely no reason to get injured, unless you're a complete moron. Learn good technique from day one, follow a decent program, and stop every set 1–2 reps shy of failure.

The point of this should be obvious. By the time you have driven yourself to failure on a movement, you've basically ignored the NFS rule *and* the rep-slowing rule. You've pushed until even your stress pathways can't help you any longer. It's likely that your form went in the toilet a few reps ago.

Stop before failure of any sort, unless you are testing or competing. Better yet, have someone watch you and stop your set for you, so you can learn the signs and signals. If every workout is a competition for you, and your honeymoon phase hasn't come to the typical crash-and-burn ending yet, come back and read this after it has.

There is a highly successful method for training that Olympic weight lifters call the "Bulgarian method." Way oversimplified, it means you will work up to a maximally heavy single rep each workout (called the "daily max") six days a week, in one or more exercises. It makes you tired and achy just thinking about it, right? Through the grapevine, however, certain important restrictions on this approach to training were lost. In his article "Maxing on Squats and Deadlifts Every Day," Greg Nuckols brought these important points up about the original Bulgarian method approach:

> Here, the daily max is a weight that you can move without mental arousal (no death metal and ammonia) and without any aberration from perfect form.

> Perfect form is imperative, though. If your squat or bench technique puts undue stress on any of your soft tissues, you'll progressively increase the damage you're inflicting rather than the benefits you're reaping.

> For someone with good form, however, the risk of injury is probably lower than it would be on other programs because you never give an all-out effort. . . .

> If you psych yourself up for your maxes every day, you'll have a greater risk of burnout, but if you approach each lift calmly (as you should), your hormonal response will probably adapt to the frequent squatting.

Note that the key points match up almost exactly with what I've already said:

+ **No psyching up**

+ **Perfect form must be maintained (stopping at face strain or rep speed slowdown would help maximize this, assuming you know what good form is)**

+ **Never give an all-out effort (go to failure)**

If it's a good enough approach for training champion Olympic weight lifters, it's good enough for you and me. Work smarter, not harder.

[5]

Breathe through your nose and don't clench your teeth.

Let's get a little evolutionary biology-ish here. What is the primary purpose of our nose? The easy answer is "breathing." If you said "smelling," consider going ten minutes without breathing and ten minutes without smelling. Are we clear now? The human nose exists to breathe. The mouth has many functions, but with regard to breathing, the mouth is a backup system and is intended only to be used in emergencies or when the nose isn't functioning correctly. In fact, one older dictionary definition of "mouth breather" is not a kind one: "a stupid person; a moron, dolt, imbecile." In the references section, I've provided a link to a website showing a significant amount of research linking negative health effects with mouth breathing.

Nasal breathing is relaxed breathing. Mouth breathing is panicked or stressed breathing. There are no relaxation techniques that involve any inhalations through the mouth, as this would be counterproductive to the goal. Are you noticing a pattern yet?

What I'm leading up to is that you should be breathing through your nose all the time—including during exercise—at minimum for the inhalations, optimally the entire breath cycle. Why? Nasal breathing is relaxing, efficient, effective for improving fitness, and health-promoting. Mouth breathing is the polar opposite of those things.

Here are some of the known benefits of nasal breathing for exercise (as opposed to mouth breathing):

+ Increases stamina and endurance

+ Prevents overtraining

+ Reduces pulse rate

+ Decreases stress on the heart

+ **Improves oxygenation of the blood**

+ **Reduces stress**

These all sound like positive effects, right?

Nasal breathing is also one of the best autoregulation tools you can use for any type of exercise. It sets a limit on how hard you can push while staying below the body's panic and stress threshold, at which point mouth breathing begins. It can also help if you don't have, or don't want to get, a heart rate monitor.

In today's world of exercise addicts and "harder is better" fitness ignorance, many will see this call for nasal breathing and say that it is impossible to create a training adaptation if you don't push hard enough to have to breathe through your mouth. Well, the best endurance runners on the planet and the research into exercise physiology beg to differ.

The Tarahumara natives of Mexico, made famous in the book *Born to Run* and renowned for their long-distance-running ability, breathe only through their noses while running, although some will exhale through a partially open mouth.

With regard to the ability to get a "training effect" from nasal breathing, in the study "Comparison of Maximal Oxygen Consumption with Oral and Nasal Breathing," researchers found that:

> While breathing through the nose only, all subjects could attain a work intensity great enough to produce an aerobic training effect (based on heart rate and percentage of VO_2 max).

Another study, "Arterial Oxygen Saturation and Peak VO_2 during Nasal and Oral Breathing," found that during treadmill running, mouth breathing resulted in only a 14 percent higher VO_2, and half of that was attributed to the higher breathing rate achievable through mouth breathing. No significant difference was found in the percentage of oxygen saturation between mouth and nasal breathing! These minimal differences won't restrict training adaptations. Just ask the Tarahumara.

Here's a personal example. I used to enjoy road cycling on my fixed-gear bike. (I've since stopped due to multiple considerations, including lack of time, pollution, bad drivers, and becoming a parent.) My main ride was from my house to my parents'— about thirty minutes each way. The hills were long and tough—so tough that time trials have been held on the longer hills. Wearing my heart rate monitor, breathing in only through my nose and out through my mouth, I was able to reach a heart rate of 170 beats per minute while really grinding out pedal strokes (fixed-gear bikes have only one gear, so there is no shifting to an easier gear on hills). Not too shabby, and definitely well above the range needed for an aerobic workout.

Here's how to breathe (chuckle). Inhale in through your nose only, and exhale out through your nose only. Do this all day, every day, and especially when you exercise. As you get into higher levels of exertion, you may have to breathe out through your mouth, just continue breathing in through your nose. Switch to inhaling through your mouth only if you are testing or in competition.

You might argue, "Well, I have a stuffy nose *all* the time and I can't breathe through my nose when I'm sitting down, much less when I'm exercising!" Here are a couple of things you can try if that is the case.

+ Apply pressure to the roof of your mouth with your tongue, which helps to open up the sinuses. To find the right spot, put your tongue behind your front upper teeth, then slide it backwards until you find that spot where your tongue sort of drops into a nice depression. Push your tongue upwards in that spot. See if this facilitates easier nasal breathing.

+ Seat yourself comfortably and, after completing a normal exhalation, pinch your nose and hold your breath while nodding your head up and down at a moderate pace (don't rush this). Hold your breath as long as possible, but not to the point where you're gasping for air. When you get an urgent desire to breathe, release your nose and take a breath. You must now remember to breathe only through your nose! Make your inhalations gentle and relax into your exhalations. After this exercise, your goal is to breathe less than before, with an increased level of relaxation. (You may breathe more for one or two minutes after holding your breath, but this should resolve itself naturally.)

+ Finally, start really paying attention to how your body reacts to foods. You may notice that certain foods create a lot of phlegm, mucus, and general sinus congestion. This will obviously make it more difficult to breathe through the nose. Over time, as I have incorporated into my daily routine many of the metabolism-increasing and stress-reducing techniques that we cover in this book, I've found that my sinus and phlegm reactions to foods have nearly disappeared—except for my reaction to gluten. My nose plugs up incredibly fast if I eat a lot of gluten, and I also tend to snore when I have it at dinner or later (snoring can be caused by nasal congestion forcing one to mouth-breathe). I take this heavily into account when I'm working out the next day. Bad sleep and plugged-up nasal passages do not make for a good workout, or a happy wife!

If you have anatomical problems that make it difficult for you to breathe through your nose, I highly recommend investigating the following devices:

http://www.normalbreathing.com/l-mouth-taping.php
www.nosebreathe.com
www.faceformer.com
www.liptrainer.com/

Look smarter, be smarter: Breathe through your nose all the time.

Moving on to teeth clenching while exercising—it's just not a good idea. While certain studies have shown that teeth clenching may result in improved short-term strength or power, this is likely due to the clenching indirectly increasing stress hormone output. Clenching and grinding the teeth while sleeping is often noted in stressed-out people, and stimulant drugs that increase adrenaline release often cause grinding and clenching. We do not want our workouts to increase our stress hormone load! In summary, during your workouts, sleep, *and* the rest of your day, your tongue should be on the roof of your mouth with your teeth slightly apart. Simple.

PART

4

SLEEP
AND
RECOVERY

Dr. Garrett Smith

Chapter 21
INTRODUCTION

Sleep and health go hand in hand—when one suffers, so does the other. There is no way around this. From my own clinical experience, I know that sleep quality and quantity are generally abysmal in developed countries. Sleep is the main "recovery" part of our day, so you will always be shortchanging your health when you don't get enough or it is of poor quality. Always prioritize fixing your sleep patterns over any other recovery approach.

This part will go beyond the more simplistic sleeping tips like "absolutely no light in your bedroom" and provide solutions that may be new to you. I won't be recommending expensive, high-tech recovery gizmos like hyperbaric chambers, body-cooling gloves, and sleep monitors. Actually, much of what I will cover is very anti-gizmo. The goal is to get back to the basics.

As described previously in Part One: Stress, the biggest difference between contemporary day-to-day life and that of previous generations (go as far back as you wish, then come up to even one or two generations before ours), which has taken a negative toll on our health as a whole, does *not* involve our diet or exercise in general. We can find people thriving in many places on foods that we may have convinced ourselves (usually based on something someone told us, not our own experience) are unhealthy, and modern exercise is a relatively new concept compared to lifestyles that simply incorporated lots of low-intensity movement throughout the day.

Our apparent lack of health in current times, in comparison to our ancestors, cannot be explained solely by our modern diets. We can find people thriving in many places on heavy consumption of foods that we may have convinced ourselves are "unhealthy." Check out the books *The Blue Zones* and *Nutrition* and *Physical Degeneration* for examples of large groups of people thriving long term on decidedly non-Paleo foods.

What is the biggest change, then? The thing that has drastically changed is our daily environment and how we interact with it throughout the day:

+ **We spend most of our time indoors.**

+ **We spend most of our time sitting.**

+ **We are separated from the ground and earth by rubber-soled shoes and nonconductive flooring (wood, plastic, vinyl).**

+ **We are continually exposed to massive human-made electro-magnetic fields (EMFs).**

+ **Our brains are constantly "on task."**

I am not interested in romanticizing the lives of our ancestors. Nor do I want to dismiss the benefits of modern society. That being said, research is increasingly showing that doing the direct opposite of the items on the above list provides immediate and tangible benefits to our health. In order to achieve these benefits, we must modify how and where we spend our time, the positions in which we spend our time, the things we interact with, and how and what we think about throughout the day.

Too many people believe that to get healthier they need to *add things* to their lives—I'm talking here about the buy-this-new-product-to-improve-your-life vision promoted by marketers. This chapter will definitely emphasize the opposite idea: To obtain health we must *remove* obstacles; we must simplify.

If some of the information in this section strikes you as a little "woo-woo" or "hippy-ish," that's fine with me. When something makes intuitive sense to me, has positive anecdotal reports that are supported by research, and fits with evolutionary biology concepts, I'll usually give it a try. Nothing ventured, nothing gained! Remember that I live in this modern world with you, and because of that, I've made sure to include only modalities and techniques that easily fit into busy schedules and lives without much intrusion or investment.

Chapter 22

GROUNDING
(EARTHING)

Until relatively recently, humans were in daily contact with the bare earth. An alien observing us now might think that we actually go out of our way to avoid touching the ground. Is it possible that a significant portion of many of our modern health issues could be a result of this disconnect between our skin and the ground, a lack of synchronization of energies between the earth and us?

However far back you choose to believe we humans have existed, for the vast majority of that time we walked, sat, stood, and slept on the ground. When our skin touches the ground, there is a real and measurable transfer of electrical energy from the earth to our body. Because we now sleep in beds and sit in chairs and wear rubber-soled shoes, we are rarely part of this "ground circuit."

A lack of connection with this ground circuit can cause electrical consequences that we are all familiar with. It's called *static electricity*. When we are insulated from the ground—typically through our rubber-soled shoes—and conditions are right, we can build up an electrical charge through a transfer of electrons that happens when certain materials are rubbed together. When the charge gets high enough and we come close to a large electrical conductor, we experience that familiar static electric shock that can be felt, heard, and seen as the excess charge is neutralized. This is an example of a negative consequence that comes about when our bodies are not grounded. While it is usually only mildly uncomfortable for us, did you know that such a static shock could damage sensitive electronics? The electricity within us is not inconsequential!

As B. Blake Levitt wrote in *Electromagnetic Fields:*

We are very slowly—some say too slowly—beginning to undergo a paradigm shift in Western medical thinking from a chemical-mechanistic model of the human body to a more finely tuned electrical-system model.

I don't want to lose people by getting too technical, and it's not really necessary. Here's what I will tell you about grounding/earthing: Our ancestors did it, the research on it is very promising, and my personal experience with it has been positive. Here's why reconnecting with the earth—touching the ground regularly, as part of your day—makes sense to me.

When an electrical system is grounded, it allows the earth to deliver or absorb electrons as needed. This avoids the buildup of electrical charges in the system that could be damaging—static electricity is an example. By grounding yourself ("earthing"), you immediately equalize your body to the same energy level, or potential, as the earth. The results of this equalization include synchronizing your internal biological clock, hormonal cycle, and physiological rhythms. Think of it as the electrical version of the synchronization that we do with the earth, as opposed to the solar, light-based version of synchronization that we do with the sun.

Research on grounding's effects on various health conditions has been conducted for over a decade now, and the following benefits have been seen:

+ Improved sleep

+ Normalized cortisol rhythms

+ Improved heart rate variability (HRV)

+ Decreased recovery time from exercise-induced delayed onset muscle soreness (DOMS)

+ Reduced blood viscosity, a major factor in cardiovascular disease

+ Reduced inflammatory markers

+ Reduced pain

With all these benefits, you're probably wondering where the sales pitch is, right? While there are earthing items that can be purchased, nothing *has* to be bought.

Here's how you can get "grounded":

+ Get your bare feet or other bare skin in contact with the ground and maintain it for at least thirty minutes. This can be done standing, walking, sitting, or lying down.

    > Surfaces that work: grass, sand, gravel, or unpainted concrete that is in contact with the earth below it.

    > Surfaces that *don't* work: wood, asphalt, carpet, or plastic.

    > If you aren't sure if your surface is grounded, test it with a body voltage meter. Through testing, I have found that the tile in my home (which is on top of concrete) is a good ground surface.

    > There are anecdotal reports that grounding for thirty minutes after a long flight will reduce or eliminate jet lag.

+ Options for shoes that allow for easy grounding:

    > EarthRunners sandals

    > ESD (ElectroStatic Discharge) shoes. These are normal-looking shoes and the most conventional option. They are available in a variety of styles.

    > ESD straps or heel grounders. These go on the outside of your shoes, connecting you to the ground via a conductive strap that touches your skin under your shoe or sock.

+ Use one or more of the Earthing™ products (available from www.earthing.com) to ground yourself inside your home and office. I highly recommend the bedsheet setups since they give multiple hours of continuous exposure at the time when you can use it most. I use the half-sheet setup at home and really notice a difference when I sleep without it. I plan to switch to the full bottom sheet option next, simply because it will stay in place better.

> The best ground source to use with any Earthing™ product is a corded ground rod that is routed into the ground outside your home. Some people report that using ground outlets in their home electrical system is less effective than a true outdoor ground connection.

One important note: Grounding may not be beneficial if there are large electrical fields around. Here's a personal example: At work I have a laptop that does not have a ground wire on its power cord (this is a bad thing, as I'll explain). While writing this book and spending lots of time at the computer, I started feeling a tingle on the back of my head while I was using it. I also noticed that I was getting very tired, irritable, and emotional by the end of the day. I decided to run a test. Using my body voltage meter, I measured the voltage while I was touching the laptop against the voltage when I was just sitting in my chair (which registered minimal ambient voltage readings). The results were *shocking* (ba-dum-tish!). When I was touching my laptop's surface, the body voltage meter showed nine volts. When my laptop was sitting on top of a leather desktop cover that had a metal core, it went up to twelve volts! For you iPad lovers, testing has revealed that the device sends up to twenty volts (ack!) through the user via the touchscreen when it is plugged in. With new theories that amyotrophic lateral sclerosis (ALS, aka Lou Gehrig's disease) could be the result of excessively administered electrically based medical treatments (including the physical therapy, athletic training, and chiropractic favorite electrical muscle stimulation, aka EMS, which have electrodes that make your muscles twitch and jump involuntarily), I'd personally rather pass on running double-digit voltages through myself for a large chunk of the day.

Based on how I felt, I suspected that running those voltages through me was not a good idea. My first idea was to make a ground cord, connect it to the grounded wall outlet, and then ground myself by holding it. I thought that if I grounded myself, my situation would improve. It did *not*. I actually felt worse . . . and confused. After more research, I figured out why. Electricity always searches for the shortest route to the ground. When I wasn't grounded, the electricity had to search for another route. Since I normally wear rubber-soled shoes, I was not the shortest route. However, once I grounded myself with the ground cord and then touched the laptop, I immediately became the shortest path to the ground and felt even worse. After this learning experience, I started grounding all my electronics *first*. There are prefab grounding cords for sale at places like www.LessEMF.com, or you can make your own. Currently, I ground my laptop via a cord connecting the wall ground outlet and one of the screws in the laptop's metal frame. The body voltage meter no longer shows an elevated reading, and my head tingling is gone (sadly, I wasn't turning into Spider-Man). In short, if you start grounding and you feel worse, either your ground connection has issues or you have unwittingly become part of a circuit that you don't want any part of. Stop doing it, step back, and figure out the problem.

We may never know how or why grounding works. It just does. Recognize that we are bioelectrical beings inhabiting an electrical planet, and get reconnected.

Chapter 23
FOREST BATHING
("GET YOUR BUTT OUTSIDE")

Hopefully, you're in touch with your body enough to know that, in general, the more time you spend outside, the better you feel. When you think about your perfect restorative and relaxing vacation, does it involve going somewhere with pleasant weather and beautiful scenery? This is your body asking you to spend time outside.

Your body instinctively knows that being outside is good for you. Yet, how much effort are you putting into actually getting out there? I'm not referring to walking from your house to your car and then from your car to your office; this does not count. Seriously, I know people who think they get enough healthy sun exposure this way!

Forest bathing is a fancy term for simply spending time in nature. It's a translation of a Japanese term, *shinrin-yoku,* and is a recognized form of stress management and relaxation in Japan. Amazingly, studies are finding all sorts of health marker improvements as a result of spending time outdoors (in forests, in particular). These include:

+ Decreased blood glucose and hemoglobin A1c values in diabetics

+ Decreased sympathetic (fight-or-flight) nervous system activity, including reductions in adrenaline and cortisol

+ Decreased blood pressure

+ Decreased feelings of hostility and depression

+ Reduced oxidative stress and inflammatory markers

+ Enhanced human natural killer (NK) cell activity and expression of anticancer proteins

+ Increased immunoglobulin A, G, and M

+ Improved mood, vigor, and liveliness

+ Increased heart rate variability, associated with improved parasympathetic ("rest and digest") nervous system activity

Several of these studies have involved relatively short exposures to the forest, such as leisurely forty-minute walks. The positive results have been shown to last days, even up to a week, from a single session.

I currently live in the southern Arizona desert, which is not exactly the middle of a forest. It's a ninety-minute round-trip drive to get to the nearest one. Am I out of luck? Hardly. Forest bathing researchers have noted positive benefits in subjects that simply watched video of a forest! My interpretation of this is that the interaction of one or more of our senses with nature is what provides the benefits. While there may be specific benefits to forest bathing, there is plenty of benefit to be derived from nearly any outdoor environment as well. Nature is the key ingredient.

Let me add a personal anecdote. The process of writing this book, in the midst of my normal life stressors, added enough stress that my sleep was negatively impacted at times. In the midst of a multiday run of poor sleep, I decided to put the "Get your butt outside to relieve stress" theory to the test. I had two free hours in the middle of the day, and the weather was great. I took my lunch to a nearby park and enjoyed it without any rush. I then came back to my office building, which has a nice, large open-air atrium with benches and palm trees. I lay down on a bench and spent some time staring up at the palm leaves blowing in the wind and then some time relaxing with my eyes shut. That night I slept more soundly than I had in a while. Coincidence? Not in my opinion.

Maybe you already exercise outdoors. You're on the right track! In a study titled "Does Participating in Physical Activity in Outdoor Natural Environments Have a Greater Effect on Physical and Mental Wellbeing than Physical Activity Indoors?" it was found that a single session of running outside in an outdoor environment (compared to the same run done indoors) provided greater feelings of revitalization, positive engagement, and increased energy, as well as decreases in tension, confusion, anger, and depression. Study participants who exercised outdoors also reported a greater inclination to repeat the activity in the future.

One important point to remember: In the Japanese forest bathing studies, the participants were taking relaxing walks or simply standing in the forest. No one was doing wind sprints or kettlebell swings! Hopefully, at this point in the book, you are realizing that a high-stress workout done in a low-stress environment might negate many of the positive effects experienced in the forest bathing studies. This is most likely because the benefits of being outside mainly stem from a reduction of stress in the body.

Maybe this is all obvious to you and the idea that being outside is good and necessary for humans to be healthy evokes an enthusiastic "Duh!" Good for you. Now walk the talk and put that knowledge to use, if you haven't already. Spread the word to others.

Being outside in nature positively impacts major aspects of our health, particularly in reducing stress hormones and improving our immune function. Spending time outside—it doesn't get more Paleo than that!

Chapter 24

ELECTROMAGNETIC FIELDS (EMFS) AND RADIO FREQUENCY RADIATION (RFR)

Want deeper, more restful sleep? Want to be happier? Want your kids to behave better? Want to reduce your risk of cancer? Want higher testosterone levels? Keep reading.

Since you live in the modern world, I'm going to bet that you willingly use a variety of (extremely non-Paleo!) devices in your house all day, every day. What you might not know is that research has indicated that these gadgets may be associated with:

+ Lower testosterone

+ DNA damage and gene changes

+ Sperm count reduction and abnormalities

+ Infertility

+ Fatigue

+ Headaches

+ Concentration difficulties

+ Increased risk of leukemia

+ Increased cancer risk

+ Sleep problems and reduced REM sleep

+ Impaired nervous system activity and neurological symptoms

+ Cardiovascular symptoms

+ Emotional changes and depression

+ Decreased cognition and memory

+ Behavioral problems and learning difficulties in children

+ Increased stress hormones

+ Decreased dopamine levels

+ Pathological leakage of the blood-brain barrier

+ Decreased immune function

+ Slowed motor skills

+ Cell membrane alterations

You might be thinking, "What the hell? Why didn't my Paleo blog guru tell me about this?" Maybe he did and you ignored it. Maybe he doesn't believe it himself.

The above list is a compilation of negative effects noted in studies done on radio frequency radiation (RFR), one of the many types of electromagnetic fields (EMFs). For most people, RFR includes things like your Wi-Fi (*anything* that is "wireless-capable," including modems, routers, computers, game systems, and DVD players); cell phones and smartphones; digital cordless telephones; digital cordless baby monitors; "smart" utility meters; and cell phone towers or antenna arrays.

Paleosphere bloggers may debate whether or not certain things are truly Paleo. What isn't up for debate is that Paleolithic folk didn't utilize electricity, wireless electronics, or have to deal with human-made EMFs. Of course, naturally occurring EMFs have always been, and will always be, present—that's not the point here. What I'm talking about are the human-made EMFs that saturate our lives in orders of magnitude greater than anything our pre-electricity and prewireless ancestors experienced.

Some of the wireless addicts reading this are getting antsy now and pulling out the old "Research doesn't say there is a problem!" line. Let me remind you of the infamous cover-ups perpetrated on the public by the corporate tobacco and asbestos industries. These cover-ups shortened many people's lives, particularly when it came to cancer. It is extremely difficult to pinpoint any one cause of cancer, mainly because of how long cancers take to develop before being found. Once the research caught up, the cause and effect became obvious. The problem is that catching up takes decades. The United States seems to be particularly beholden to corporations, whose representatives have a history of suppressing research contrary to their interests. That's likely why I remember hearing a statement years ago that the only country not producing study data that cellular and wireless technologies cause health issues was the good ol' US of A.

Paleo followers have known for years that the policies of government agencies are often guided and driven by corporations only concerned about their profits (the USDA with nutrition and the FDA with pharmaceuticals, for instance). Safety is not a concern for these corporate sharks; more money is. Maybe you're one of those eternal optimists who want to trust the government and believe these agencies have your best interests at heart. That's cute; it's like children believing in Santa Claus.

There are essentially two camps at work when it comes to RFR and EMFs. One is composed of researchers, scientists, electrosensitive people (those whose health and quality of life suffer from exposure to EMFs), and other intelligent, open-minded people who follow the "precautionary principle" and wonder if any of these new technologies could be harmful. The other camp, as usual, consists of well-funded lobbyists schmoozing government agencies and their corporate sponsors.

Let's start looking more deeply at the latter camp, their members, and their stances. First, they deny there are negative health effects from RFR at all. To relate this camp to another current health issue and how our government agencies are dealing with it—maybe you've heard of Monsanto? Maybe you have a strong visceral reaction to that word based on what you already know about their products. Maybe you aren't so sure that human health and safety are considerations for them at all. Could the same be true for other corporations, too? You should know that Michael Taylor, the current deputy commissioner of the Food and Drug Administration (FDA), was formerly the

Monsanto vice president for public policy. Not a good sign, if you ask me.

On that note, what does the FDA have to say about RFR? From the FDA.gov website:

> Many people are concerned that cell phone radiation will cause cancer or other serious health hazards. **The weight of scientific evidence has not linked cell phones with any health problems.** (emphasis mine)

Now what does the Federal Communications Commission (FCC—the government agency in charge of regulating interstate and international communications by radio, television, wire, cellular, satellite, and cable) say about RFR and human health? From the FCC.gov website:

> Some health and safety interest groups have interpreted certain reports to suggest that wireless device use may be linked to cancer and other illnesses, posing potentially greater risks for children than adults. While these assertions have gained increased public attention, **currently no scientific evidence establishes a causal link between wireless device use and cancer or other illnesses.** (emphasis mine)

I was always taught not to use absolute terms, because once a single exception is found, it undermines the whole argument. Saying there is *no* scientific evidence is a very strong statement, and the FDA and the FCC seem to be on the same page regarding this statement. Your government is basically saying, "Trust us, move along, nothing to see here!"

Before we begin punching holes in this claim, recall the asbestos and tobacco industry cover-ups that caused many, many people to get sick and die over decades (in the case of asbestos, it was more than a century before the government was forced to admit that this substance caused problems) before laws were finally enacted to protect people. Both industries spent huge sums of money to produce bogus research and influence lawmakers so that the corporations making these products could sell more of them. To see this psychopathic approach documented, look for the article "Tobacco Explained: The Truth about the Tobacco Industry . . . in Its Own Words" on the World Health Organization website.

The more money there is at stake, the more an industry will work to protect itself, human health be damned. So let's get an idea of how much money is involved here. Electronics (business and consumer) is a billion-dollar, if not trillion-dollar, industry. Apple Inc. alone had worldwide revenues of $156 billion in 2012; Verizon's worldwide revenues came in at around $116 billion that same year. That's just two of the myriad companies in the electronics and wireless industry. To put this in perspective: Total revenue for the entire tobacco industry worldwide for 2012 was $670 billion. I'm going to go out on a limb and assume that the electronics and wireless industries as a whole earned much more than that in a year. And with money comes influence.

After seeing those numbers, you tell me if you think the electronics and wireless industries have some vested interest in hiding the truth about how their products may negatively impact the health of those who use them. I'd also venture to say that many of you probably don't want to hear that your favorite electronic leash or distraction gadget is slowly ruining your health. Ignorance is bliss, they say . . . until it isn't. Don't get me wrong; I think people should do whatever the hell they want, as long as what they choose isn't harming others. Therein lies the problem with EMF. You don't get a choice. Walls don't block them; they cannot be seen, touched, smelled, or heard. They're like secondhand smoke in that we have no choice when it comes to limiting our exposure, precisely because we can't tell where they are (without a meter).

Moving on, over to the side that disputes the government's claims that there is no evidence that RFR and EMFs cause any health problems. What if this side had quite a bit of research (as in, "scientific evidence") linking EMFs of various types with multiple health issues? Wouldn't this quickly poke major holes in the government agencies' claims that there are no negative health issues related to EMFs?

The BioInitiative Report (www.bioinitiative.org) came out in 2007 and was updated in 2012. The following quotes are from both the report itself and the website.

What is it: A report by 29 independent scientists and health experts from around the world about possible risks from wireless technologies and electromagnetic fields. . . .

The great strength of the BioInitiative Report is that it has been done independent of governments, existing bodies and industry professional societies that have clung to old standards. Precisely because of this, the BioInitiative Report presents a solid scientific and public health policy assessment that is evidence-based. . . .

What it covers: The science, public health, public policy and global response to the growing health issue of chronic exposure to electromagnetic fields and radiofrequency radiation in the daily life of billions of people around the world. **Covers brain tumor risks from cell phones, damage to DNA and genes, effects on memory, learning, behavior, attention; sleep disruption and cancer and neurological diseases like Alzheimer's disease. Effects on sperm and miscarriage (fertility and reproduction), effects of wireless on the brain development of the fetus and infant, and effects of wireless classrooms on children and adolescents is addressed.** Mechanisms for biological action and public health responses in other countries are discussed. Therapeutic use of very low intensity EMF and RFR are addressed. . . .

Roughly, **1,800 new studies have been published in the last five years** reporting effects at exposure levels ten to hundreds or thousands of times lower than allowed under safety limits in most countries of the world. (emphasis mine)

It's strange that the FDA and FCC have no access to these *1,800 studies* released since 2007, or to the evidence that supports the EMF-related health problems that I listed at the start of this chapter (compiled from the well-referenced "RF Color Charts" on the BioInitiative Report website). The entire BioInitiative Report covers over 2,000 research studies on various forms of EMFs and observed effects on human and animal health. That's quite a weighty pile of information that the government has been sweeping under the carpet!

Wait, there's more! The Environmental Working Group (www.EWG.org) is this country's leading environmental health research and advocacy organization. You may be familiar with its lists of the best and worst fruits and vegetables to eat with regard to pesticide residues. They've also created an executive summary about the researched risks of cell phone use. Here are some of their main points:

Scientists have known for decades that high doses of the radiofrequency radiation emitted by cell phones can penetrate the body, heat tissues, trigger behavioral problems and damage sensitive tissues like the eyeball and testicle. . . .

Yet when cell phones went on the market in the 1980s, federal regulators did not require manufacturers to prove they were safe. . . .

In response to the growing debate over the safety of cell phone emissions, government agencies in Germany, Switzerland, Israel, United Kingdom, France, and Finland and the European Parliament have recommended actions to help consumers—especially young children—reduce their exposure to cell phone radiation.

In contrast, the two U.S. federal agencies that regulate cell phones, the Food and Drug Administration (FDA) and the Federal Communication Commission (FCC), have all but ignored evidence that long term cell phone use may be risky.

The FCC adopted radiation standards developed by the cell phone industry 17 years ago. These standards, still in use, allow

20 times more radiation to reach the head than the rest of the body. They do not account for risks to children. . . .

Current FCC standards fail to provide an adequate margin of safety for cell phone radiation exposure and lack a meaningful biological basis. . . .

Current standards provide 40 times less protection than typical government health limits for environmental exposures.

What part of the above sounds like the FCC has your health in mind? Not having to prove that cell phones are safe, seventeen-year-old standards, allowing twenty times more radiation to the head than the body, not accounting for risks to children, inadequate safety margins, lacking biological basis, forty times less protective standards than other environmental exposures. Come on.

If only there was a government agency willing to push for standards based on all the evidence. Oh, wait. The U.S. Environmental Protection Agency already tried that. For some unknown reason, the EPA's guidelines have been permanently suppressed. This is from www.electromagnetichealth.org:

Like Sisyphus eternally pushing the rock uphill, the Environmental Protection Agency tried to birth human exposure guidelines for radio frequency radiation for 17 years.

First there was opposition from other federal agencies. The FDA didn't want the exposure limits to apply to microwave ovens or VDTs. A number of agencies didn't want them to apply to occupational exposures. The FAA didn't want to have to protect the public from air traffic control and weather radars. The DoD didn't want military radars to be affected. In 1987, EPA terminated its microwave health effects research program, and in 1988 suspended the development of its exposure guidelines for a third time.

But Senator Joseph Lieberman convened Congressional hearings in 1992, inquiring into an epidemic of testicular cancer in policemen who used traffic radar guns. These hearings resulted in renewed pressure put on EPA by various members of Congress to resume its work. Finally in June 1995, E. Ramona Trovato, Director of the Office of Radiation and Indoor Air, announced that the guidelines were substantially complete and would be issued "in early 1996."

This time EPA's efforts were on a collision course with plans for ubiquitous cell phone service. For the new guidelines stated explicitly that they protected only against shocks and burns and the effects of RF heating and did "not apply to chronic, nonthermal exposure situations." EPA further announced that it was ready to proceed to Phase 2 of its regulatory process, which would address chronic exposure and non–thermal effects and take an additional two years. **Cell phones would have been illegal, but for one circumstance: EPA's exposure guidelines have never seen the light of day.** (emphasis mine)

The FDA and the FCC are like the proverbial bullies kicking sand in the wimpy EPA's face. Shameful.

When I start talking to people who can't believe that their laptops, tablets, cell phones, or nearby cell towers could be harming them, I ask if they've observed any of the following:

+ **Warming of the ear and head after talking on the cell phone for extended periods. Most people understand this best when I liken it to microwaving your brain, because that's actually what's happening!**

+ **Poor sleep when their cell phones, laptops, tablets, wireless modems, or any other wireless-capable items are within close range (six feet) of their head while in bed. This sleep state is often described as not feeling like they are ever getting into deep sleep; it is a more superficial state of sleep often punctuated with many awakenings. Another version of it is when** people simply never drop into sleep at all, yet their mind is generally quiet as they lie awake all night. Some note that they even seem to feel a mild buzzing inside their head.

+ Feeling the area where they normally keep their phone vibrate when their phone isn't there.

+ Tinnitus (ringing in the ears) when using a cellular or cordless phone.

+ Salivary gland problems on the side of the head where they typically use their cell phone.

+ Decrease in visual ability. This is often noticed immediately after looking at a screen for extended periods.

These are early signs of a developing electrosensitivity (some call it electrohypersensitivity). Trust me, you want to stop this process early, because not addressing it will only make it worse! Sadly, much like chronic smokers, most people won't take action until they realize (or admit) the connection between EMFs and their symptoms. Recovery can only begin once their environment is thoroughly cleaned of most, if not all, major sources of EMFs.

I started paying attention to this information the first time my ear and head got hot from using a cell phone back in 1994. More alarming was when I felt the area under my pants pocket, the place where I typically carried my cell phone, vibrate when I wasn't carrying it. Without knowing anything technical about EMFs at all, I knew that those were bad signs. If all this is making you think twice about EMFs and you're looking for ways to take action, check out the next chapter.

So what are these EMFs actually doing to our bodies to potentially cause so many different health issues? Here are the major processes discovered in the research:

+ Creating interference in normal electrical communication between cells. This could disrupt cellular function anywhere and everywhere within the body, negatively impacting sleep, hormone production, brain function, immune function, and healing (regenerative) functions.

+ Reducing melatonin production. This neurohormone and antioxidant is critical to sleep and protecting cells from genetic damage.

+ Creating a state of chronic inflammation in the body, including causing the release of proinflammatory substances like histamines and cytokines as part of a protective mechanism.

+ Overstimulating the immune system initially, then suppressing it over the long term.

+ Raising cortisol and adrenaline levels, affecting sleep, immunity (and therefore autoimmunity), cardiovascular function, premature aging, and more.

+ Locking cell membranes into an inactive state, preventing the release of toxins and free radicals. This may lead to DNA damage and a reduced ability to heal, both thought to be early steps on the road to development of cancer.

+ Causing calcium ion efflux from the cells. This may be linked to neurological degeneration, cancer, heart arrhythmias, and more.

+ Elevating blood sugar and blood viscosity (that is, making thicker blood), both of which increase risk of cardiovascular disease.

Many Paleo followers have lost faith in government organizations and private industry to properly inform them with regard to nutrition and other health-related issues. Why in the world would you trust them on this?

So how do we clean up the EMFs from our living and working spaces? This is where things get tough.

The Perfect Health Cluster

Matt Stone

Whoa, whoa, whoa, Garrett, buddy! I thought we talked about this! You said we weren't going to write a book that was going to make people want to retreat into the wilderness to wear loincloths and try to be hunter-gatherers! Although your wife did mention something about wanting to see you adorned in such a garment. Hey, it's hot in Arizona. You could pull it off in Sedona, no doubt (too many cacti in Tucson, though—yikes!).

I started out with a "move to a deserted island" fantasy in the back of my head when I first encountered a lot of negative information about our modern world. From genetically modified food to getting zapped with invisible frickin' laser beams, many times it seemed the only reasonable solution to modern problems was not to be modern. I made this a near-reality on many occasions. I feel lucky that I'm not the guy in Moab who lives in a cave and comes down from the hills from time to time to update his blog at the public library. No, really, this guy does exist. No, it's not me. Nice try.

One of the authors on my site, Rob Archangel, came up with a great reminder about health pursuits: "Persistence is better than perfection." So is progress.

I, too, have broached this subject elsewhere, drawing parallels between dietary perfectionism and the use of global resources. Hey, just because it's a problem to abuse electricity and fossil fuels doesn't mean we should trade in our car for a Schwinn and live by candlelight. A 50 percent reduction in consumption is significant and allows you to function like a normal person. The same goes for eating. Just because wheatgrass juice is nutritious and Coca-Cola isn't doesn't mean you have to drink only wheatgrass juice and never, ever touch a soft drink. Drink less soda and eat more nutritious foods. Your nutrition doesn't have to be 100 percent perfection. It's not an all-or-nothing kind of thing.

I bring this up here as Garrett informs us of what I fully believe based on my own research and personal experience (laptop directly on lap equals blue balls, aching knees, and horrid body odor) to be extremely important information about our health. But there is absolutely no reason to run to the Verizon store and cancel your phone contract and start sleeping on the ground in your backyard. I hope most of you do not need this kind of reminder, but in my experience dealing with people who devour health books and websites the way the rest of the world gobbles up sleeves of Thin Mints, the tendency to become paralyzed by the pursuit of perfection is very real and very common.

Do not allow yourself to become victimized, "hermitized," and paralyzed by health information of any kind. Paying attention to your health should be about enhancing your life, not obliterating it. Your health practices need to take your social life into account, your professional life into account, your family life into account, your bank account into account (hey, I figured if I was going to be redundant why do it half-assed?), and more. Once you've assessed all those things and thought about your own personal priorities, pick your battles, and hopefully make any changes in a moderate, sane, and practical way.

Life is too short and the modern world is too cool to isolate yourself. Use this information, as well as any health information, to make your life better. If all you can reasonably do is sleep with your phone in Airplane Mode and out of your bedroom, you are already way ahead of everyone else. I just wrote the last two sentences with the Wi-Fi turned off on my laptop, and it's sitting on a table instead of my crotch. That's good enough for me. Do you have any gold stars or badges for me, Garrett?

Make some little changes and do it in a confident, empowered, and informed way. This chapter is not bad news or more downer, depressive info about the world we live in. It's great, and Garrett provides clear, easy action steps that involve simple changes in your daily habits. I know I needed the reminder, and odds are you did, too.

Remember, too, that the human psyche is capable of experiencing mental stress in just about any situation. If you hear that vegetable oil is bad for you, are you going to panic every time you eat at a restaurant, knowing what kind of oil they are using in the kitchen? If you know that Wi-Fi signals can do some damage, are you going to quit your office job and put your whole family's well-being in jeopardy by switching to a $10-an-hour job as a lifeguard at the local outdoor pool? If you do, the stress is likely to get you long before vegetable oil and EMFs ever could.

Instead, take comfort in what you *can* do, like not talking with the cell phone pressed against your ear, or cooking at home with butter and coconut oil instead of canola. You are taking action, it will make a difference, and it need not interfere with your life or cause you undue stress and worry. It may take some Jedi mind tricks to sort it out and get the benefits of your health practices without the unintended consequences of worry and stress, but you'll figure it out if you remember to make your health practices a part of your life instead of your entire life.

Chapter 25

TAKE ACTION!

Now that you know about the issues with EMFs in general, you're probably wondering what to do about it. The options are numerous, ranging from a couple of simple things I've found that help people sleep to trying to eliminate "electro-smog pollution" as much as possible from your environments.

For those of you who want the maximal benefit for minimal investment, here's the short list of what to do in your house before bed to help you sleep better (there's more info on each one to come; this is the abbreviated version):

1. Turn your cell phone to Airplane Mode or move it as far away from your bed as you can. Turn up the ringer volume as necessary when you do this.

2. Unplug all cordless phones.

3. Unplug or disable the wireless function on anything with wireless capability: modems, routers, laptops, DVD players, game systems, and so on.

4. Move anything that plugs into the wall at least six feet from where your head rests while in bed—alarm clocks, in particular! The six-foot rule includes the item itself and the cord.

I've helped entire families fix their chronic insomnia in one night with those simple suggestions. No joke! In each of the sections below, I'll begin with the *least* intrusive actions you can take to lower your EMF exposure and progress onward.

Cell Phones and Smartphones

+ Realize that cell phones are regularly "pinging" base stations—sending signals to check in—even when they aren't actively receiving phone calls, texts, or e-mails. Actively using your cell phone increases the transmissions drastically, but don't think that just because you aren't using it, nothing is happening.

+ Know that many cell phones still send and receive transmissions while they are turned off. The only way to know that a cell phone is not emitting a signal is to put it in Airplane Mode. (This is easily done; refer to your phone's manual.) I suggest people leave their phone on Airplane Mode nearly all the time, switching Airplane Mode off only to check or reply to voice mails, texts, and e-mails; once you are finished, switch Airplane Mode back on. This minimizes the EMFs sent out by your phone and doesn't significantly change how you use it, other than that someone calling your cell phone when Airplane Mode is on will go straight to voice mail. Airplane Mode makes EMF a nonissue when your phone is on, while keeping most of your phone's other capabilities available.

+ Do not sleep with your cell phone under your pillow, next to your bed, or within a minimum of six feet of your head while you are sleeping. If you have chronic insomnia or poor quality of sleep (that is, you don't wake up refreshed) and you keep your phone close to your bed, this is probably a major culprit. Nothing I've done has been more consistently effective at improving sleep quality than moving the cell phone as far away from the bed as possible. If you want to use your cell phone as an alarm and keep it close to your bed, the only setup I endorse is *not* having the phone plugged in and turning it on Airplane Mode. As I mentioned previously, just because a phone is off doesn't mean it isn't emitting EMFs. If you feel you must leave your cell phone on at night, turn up the ringer volume and put it as far away from you as possible.

+ Children are anywhere from two to ten times more suscep-
  tible than adults to the damaging effects of EMFs, due to their
  thinner skulls and smaller bodies, which allow for effectively
  deeper penetration. A cell phone is not a toy! If your kids want
  to play with apps on your phone, make sure it is on Airplane
  Mode. If your kids are going to talk on a cell phone, make sure
  to use the speakerphone so they can keep it far from the ear.

  > People who begin using cell phones as teenagers or younger
    have a 680 percent higher risk of glioma brain tumors.

  > Health agencies in six nations—Switzerland, Germany, Is-
    rael, France, the United Kingdom, and Finland—have recom-
    mended reducing children's exposures to cell phone radia-
    tion.

+ Pregnant women should not keep or hold their cell phone anywhere near their belly. If I were a pregnant woman, I would
  avoid cell phones like the plague. If you insist on using one,
  consider a product like Belly Armor (www.bellyarmor.com) to
  protect your unborn child—and then consider the cognitive
  dissonance required to admit that your cell phone is bad for
  them but somehow isn't affecting you.

  > Children who were exposed to cell phones before and just af-
    ter birth tend to have a higher prevalence of emotional symp-
    toms, behavioral problems, inattention, hyperactivity, and
    problems with peers. When children whose mothers used
    cell phones during pregnancy also used cell phones them-
    selves, they were 80 percent more likely to have behavioral
    problems, compared to children who do not use a cell phone
    and whose mothers did not use cell phones during pregnan-
    cy. When looking at cell phone use during pregnancy alone,
    children of mothers who used cell phones were 54 percent
    more likely to have behavioral problems.

+ Don't put a cell phone within six to eight inches of a pacemak-
  er, or you might have real problems—like, uh, death. Seriously.

+ Keep your cell phone a minimum of one inch away from your body at all times, unless it is in Airplane Mode. Distance is your friend with any type of EMFs!

+ Don't use your cell phone when the signal is weak. The phone will drastically increase its transmission strength to compensate.

+ Don't use your cell phone when you are surrounded by metal (for example, in a car, train, or plane). Not only is your signal weakened by having to go through the metal (thus increasing your phone's RFR output to compensate), but also the metal is reflecting much of the RFR right back onto you, multiplying your exposure. I suggest turning your phone on Airplane Mode while driving; you shouldn't be talking, texting, or e-mailing while behind the wheel anyway, right?

  > A 2010 experiment with *Car and Driver* magazine editor Eddie Alterman that took place at a deserted airstrip showed that texting while driving had a greater impact on safety than driving drunk. While he was legally drunk, Alterman's stopping distance from 70 mph increased by four feet. By contrast, reading an e-mail while sober added thirty-six feet, and sending a text added seventy feet.

+ Minimize talking on your cell phone. Use landlines with corded phones whenever possible. Text instead of talking.

+ Maximize distance between the cell phone and your head while talking. This can be done through using the speaker-phone or a headset. The air tube–wired headsets are best; the worst are wireless headsets. (Adding another EMF source is like trying to make two wrongs equal a right.)

+ If you are close to a computer (preferably with a hardlined Ethernet connection), use that computer instead of your phone for anything Internet-related.

+ If you seriously reduce your cell phone usage, consider getting a pay-as-you-go cell phone service. After getting serious about minimizing my cell phone use, I saw my monthly data usage drop by 90 percent. Why pay for something you aren't using?

+ Gadgets that claim to turn your cell phone's harmful energy into neutral, beneficial energy *do not* reduce the actual EMFs you are absorbing. If they do help, conventional EMF-measuring instruments have been unable to assess how. "Buyer beware" is all I can say. I am open to the idea that they may help, but the guaranteed safest thing to do is to reduce or eliminate your exposure. That said, the Pong Research cell phone cases have been demonstrated to focus and direct the cell phone radiation away from your head and body—toward the back side of the phone—while also improving reception, thus reducing the signal strength your phone has to transmit. They are legit.

+ The ultimate reduction in cell phone radiation exposure (and expense!) comes from getting rid of your cell phone. You've cleaned up your nutrition; why not clean up your environment? As a doctor and father of two young children, I admit that I still have a cell phone, yet it stays on Airplane Mode for 99 percent of the day.

Cordless (DECT—Digital Enhanced Cordless Telecommunications) Landline Phones

+ When using a cordless phone, use the speakerphone whenever possible and limit the time you spend on it.

+ Realize that the main base station of a cordless (DECT) phone is the major source of radiation and that it constantly emits a high amount of EMFs in a circular cloud around it.

+ Here are the landline phone options arranged in order from best to worst:

> Corded phones. Try to use these exclusively (not a corded-plus-cordless hybrid). I recently purchased a brand-new corded phone for $16. Buying multiple phones for various

rooms, along with longer cords, makes them easier to use. You may need to contact your phone company to get additional landline filters, but they are inexpensive.

> Old-style analog cordless phones. The ones with the collapsible metal antennas emit minimal EMF and are not an issue. This is not true of the cordless phones with "stubby" or nonexistent antennas.

> "Eco" DECT cordless phones. When enabled (and make sure you enable it; it isn't automatic), the "Eco" mode drastically reduces or eliminates the EMF coming from the base when the phone is docked, adjusts EMF output based on how far the phone base is from the handset (most cordless phone bases emit a constantly high amount of RFR regardless of how far the handset is from the base), reduces the RFR transmitting power in general (this reduces the effective distance from the base that the phone will still function), and reduces the electricity consumption of the phone by more than 50 percent.

> DECT cordless phones. If you continue to use a regular DECT cordless phone, unplug the base at night (get a corded phone as well to cover emergency calls) and move it far away from the areas you inhabit when it is plugged in.

Bedrooms

+ Keep plug-in alarm clocks—along with anything else that plugs into the wall (item and cord included)—at least six feet from the bed. Alarm clocks emit notoriously high EMFs and often sit close to your head while you sleep. Consider using a battery-operated alarm clock instead.

+ Move beds, cribs, and couches away from walls where your electrical wiring is located or where there is an electrical panel (fuse box) or major appliance (like a refrigerator) on the other side of the wall. A couple extra inches of distance are much better than nothing! This also goes for the floors above or below appliances or electrical panels. Do the best you can.

+ Do not use electric blankets or heating pads. Turn off water bed heaters when in bed.

+ If you have electric baseboard heaters, move beds and cribs away from them.

Wireless Internet, Modems, and Routers

+ If possible, avoid installing a wireless network in your home. Choose a hardline Ethernet connection instead. You may need a professional to come and wire your home for Ethernet. It may cost you something, but have you priced cancer treatments lately?

+ When you are not using the wireless Internet, turn it off. This is easily accomplished by doing an Internet search for "[your modem/router model] turn wireless off" and following the instructions the search reveals. Be aware that some modems will automatically turn the wireless signal back on when they receive updates.

> For non–computer savvy people, an easier solution is to simply unplug wireless modems and routers while sleeping and when not actively using them.

+ If your computer can receive a wireless signal, that means it is also emitting its own wireless signal. If you aren't actively using wireless capability, make sure to turn off the computer's wireless as well. Some computers have actual switches to turn off their internal wireless devices, while in others this is done through the computer settings.

Computers and Tablets

+ Use a corded (hardline, Ethernet) Internet connection instead of a wireless connection. You can have professionals install

Ethernet outlets at necessary locations in your home and office, or do it yourself if you are so inclined.

+ Never use a laptop computer or tablet on your lap or near your internal organs. If you use a laptop, use it on battery power as often as you can, and consider using a radiation-shielding HARApad (www.harapad.com) underneath it if you have to put it on your lap.

> *According to one study, normal sperm in a petri dish, exposed to four hours of a Wi-Fi–connected laptop, had a significant decrease in motility and an increase in DNA fragmentation (meaning the sperm were less healthy and capable of movement).*

+ Replace old computer monitors with LED or LCD models, which emit less electromagnetic radiation.

+ Turn off and unplug computers, printers, video game consoles, and other electronics when they're not in use.

Wireless-Capable Electronics

+ Turn off the wireless function when you aren't using it, especially at night. This includes cordless baby monitors, wireless DVD players, and gaming systems. If you aren't using the wireless option, turn it off! Refer to the owner's manual. I've found that if you to turn the item to "wired setup" (meaning a hardlined Ethernet cable, whether or not there is actually a cable), it will automatically turn the wireless transmission off.

+ If you don't know how to turn the wireless function off on any item, unplugging it will generally take care of that problem.

Power Cords

+ Clean them up. This is particularly important for power cords with transformers (the little rectangular box that is either on the plug or somewhere along the cord). Move them as far as possible from your feet and sitting area.

+ Minimize plug strips and surge protectors. These generally put out high EMF. Treat them like power cords. Move them as far away from your feet and sitting area as possible. Try to consolidate your plug strips—say, from two in a given area to only one.

Lights

+ Avoid installing compact fluorescent light bulbs (CFLs), fluorescent tubes, and low-voltage halogen lights. Use incandescent bulbs or LED (light-emitting diode) bulbs instead.

> *According to one study, the response of healthy skin cells to UV emitted from CFL bulbs is consistent with damage from ultraviolet radiation. Incandescent light of the same intensity had no effect on healthy skin cells.*

+ Avoid dimmer switches. Replace them with simple on/off switches. If you have to use a dimmer switch, turn it all the way up or all the way off. Don't use the midway settings.

Televisions

+ Replace older TVs and plasma TVs with LED/LCD models, which emit less electromagnetic radiation. Plasma TVs are particularly bad.

+ Do not sit closer than six feet from your TV. This goes double for your children.

Kitchen

+ Get rid of your microwave oven. If you can't live without it, only use it for reheating things (not to cook anything), and stand at least ten feet from the oven when it is operating (to the side is preferable to standing in front of it). Never let your children put their face close to a running microwave.

+ Unplug any kitchen item that is not in use.

Garage Door Opener

+ Unplug garage door openers. These devices create a standing electromagnetic field that radiates hundreds of feet.

Smart Meters

+ Short story: Wireless smart meters are being installed on electrical panels of homes and businesses to replace the older analog meters. This creates a source of electromagnetic radiation on your house that you did not request and may have great difficulty getting rid of once it is installed. People are already experiencing significant health problems as a result of these meters. Here are some things you can do to prevent illegal installation of these meters on your home.

1. First, check to see if one has been installed. If you see a digital screen (not the dials of the analog meters), you have a wireless smart meter.

2. If one has not been installed, check your electric company's website to see if they are planning future installation of smart meters.

3. Consider sending a letter to your electric company requesting they avoid installing a smart meter on your home. (Other types of utility companies are also moving toward smart meters as well.) Other methods people have used to discourage smart meter installation involve installing a meter lock and creating a weatherproof sign for their meter to ward off those who would install a smart meter on their home against their will.

4. If you already have a smart meter installed, look into shielding your home from its EMF. That is beyond the scope of this chapter,

but you can go to websites like www.electricsense.com for more information.

Home and Office Electrical Systems

+ Unplug items from the wall if they are not in use. Of less benefit is turning off items if they are not in use. In some instances, if you have multiple items on a plug strip, you can either unplug the strip or turn off its switch.

+ Turn off the electricity at the panel (fuse box) when you don't need it. For ease of use, there are remote switches that can be installed so you can turn them on and off from inside your home.

Screen Addiction

Matt Stone

Garrett talked about exercise addiction, and I would agree whole-heartedly that exercise addiction is a real thing that does operate by the mechanisms he described. I, too, was once an exercise addict. There is another type of addiction out there, too, that so many of us struggle with, myself included—the dreaded screen addiction.

Americans supposedly watch some four hours of television daily. And many of us spend our workday in front of a computer. At home, between Facebook, video games, our favorite blogs, movies, TV, and lots of attractive naked people doing fun things on the Internet, it's awfully tough to spend much time looking away from one of the glowing boxes surrounding us.

But it's very important for us to find a way to untether ourselves from these neat gadgets. I've had the privilege of experiencing life with no gadgets at all. Zilch. Nada. Until 2006, all I had was an e-mail account. I didn't even own a computer that was connected to the Internet; I hardly ever used a computer unless I had the itch to write something. I didn't have a cell phone or a television, either—I hadn't had one of those since I left home after high school. Television was something that I left behind after leaving the nest because I noticed that I watched way too much of it. I feel as if I spent the entire eighties in front of the tube. I can whip up a tremendous array of eighties pop references, but other than that I don't have much to show for that era of my life.

And, I must say, life with very few screens is totally different.

Can you imagine how completely bored you would be sitting around in your house with no television, computer, or phone? Could you sit still for three, four, five hours at a time, as you can when a screen is there to enchant you? Let me tell you, you would find something to do, and it would likely be more creative, productive, social, or active . . . and out of your house. You would reap the rewards of physical activity over sitting, the company and conversation of others, and the hormonal and psychological benefits of being outside. You would get more vitamin D—as well as stay tan year-round so that you don't get sunburned on the rare occasion that you spend several hours out—lessen your exposure to EMF tremendously, be more grounded—literally, especially with the right footwear or lack thereof—and just generally live a life with more vigor and enthusiasm.

Life away from screens is profoundly healthful, and it's much more integral to attaining the health status of a wild animal or prehistoric human than whether you get your carbohydrates from yams or grains. And even if it wasn't healthier, it would be worth it just by virtue of the fact that you would live life more creatively, socially, and adventurously—ultimately filling the canvas of your memory with richer, more diverse, and more distinct experiences.

The question is this: What's the trick to breaking free from the alluring grip of screens? If you find the answer to that one, let me know. It's a lot easier said than done. Any time you are bored, it's awfully hard not to just flip up the laptop or press the "on" button on the remote control, or grab your nifty smartphone or tablet. Real hard. And once you have reached out to satisfy that empty feeling with an electronic device, you're gone.

It's a sensitive subject. Not everyone feels the way I do about screen life. But most who see no harm in them are those who haven't gone several months at a time without having to amuse themselves in other ways. They haven't experienced the richness of life that comes with being unable to just reach out and turn something on when there appears to be nothing better to do. When there is this empty space, people fill it with things that are usually more creative and inspiring—outdoor adventures, learning how to cook great food from scratch, painting, or learning to play instruments, or even just having one of those old-fashioned, face-to-face conversations where everyone is fully attentive.

So no, I don't have the answer for how you can do it. Like everything else in this book, screen time is not something you can do away with completely, but any effort to cut back really pays off. Reduction over elimination.

Perhaps the best strategy you can employ, and what I try to do personally as best I can, is to only use screens productively. Hours can go by on YouTube or Facebook or truTV while you accomplish nothing. There are plenty of places where you can waste a hundred clicks a day on the refresh button, too. Day trading, anyone? I know certain places and certain things on the Internet that are a waste of time for me and bring me no fulfillment, and places and things on the Internet that are productive and truly do bring me a feeling of fulfillment. I do think the Internet is, without question, the most incredible learning tool ever created. Use screens to learn, have meaningful discussion, and express yourself creatively—but find that place where you draw the line and stick with it as best you can.

As I said, it's easier said than done, but hopefully this, as well as Garrett's information on EMF and RFR, will give you more inspiration to do what you probably already know you should—not because it's "bad" to be spending so much time playing video games and fiddling around, but because you want to live a better, healthier life. You know, do some shit. Be somebody.

CONCLUSION

Matt Stone

Well, there ya have it. Any questions?

Hopefully now you have a better understanding of your body and a better appreciation of its intelligence. I hope we have given you some good ideas and encouraged you to make positive, healthful changes in your life.

While your first reaction to this book might be to feel a little directionless, or feel that the book is missing a little something since we don't give you an easy-to-follow prescription, in time you will find the tiniest of things in here to be very powerful. Take the simple idea to "eat for heat," for instance. Once you start paying even the slightest amount of attention to things like your urine concentration, the warmth of your hands and feet, and your body temperature, never again will you be able to knowingly participate in metabolically harmful dietary or exercise practices. You will immediately recognize the metabolic warning signs and stop.

How about when you feel stiff, tired, and irritable from a long day working on the computer? Will you become more aware of your body and mood? Will you take notice of the outdoor strolls and warm baths that make you feel completely different and start choosing those more regularly?

Or what about when you really push hard at the gym, can't sleep that night, and get sick the next day? Will you heed those warnings and start to exercise in a way that enhances your health and is within your stress threshold? Or is CT Fletcher right and overtraining is "just a myth perpetuated by weaklings afraid of workin' hard"? I don't think so, and I hope we proved otherwise.

The bottom line? We are smart creatures. I don't mean "smart" in the sense that we can do algebra, but "smart" in the sense that our biological template is hardwired with millennia of fine-tuned information regarding the maintenance of proper function. It manifests in observable feelings like stiffness, restlessness, yawning, burning sensations in our eyes, hunger, thirst, cravings, fullness, muscle soreness, pain, sexual desire, and happiness (just to name a few).

We are in a completely new era of human civilization. The information age we now live in might be well-intentioned, but it's drowning out our greatest source of health information: our bodies. Information and scientific study have clearly benefited us tremendously, and they should help to guide our food and lifestyle choices. They should guide whether or not we wear shoes with rubber or leather soles. They should guide whether we use Wi-Fi or an Ethernet cable to do computer work. But information and scientific study are not everything, and we must be cognizant of inner cues first, outside information second.

Let me make it easy for you and boil this book down to an easy-to-remember list.

+ Assess your total stress load and make some adjustments to lessen it.

+ Improve your Metabolism Report Card with some minor dietary tweaks, such as more salt, carbohydrates, calories, gelatin, and saturated fat, and less polyunsaturated fat (LA and AA) and muscle meat.

+ Get more sleep, and take a few simple steps to improve your sleep, like removing electronic devices and cords from your sleeping area.

+ Modify your exercise routine so that it is less stressful, and spend less time sitting.

+ Spend more time outside.

+ Increase the time you spend grounded.

+ **Take some action to reduce your exposure to EMFs and RFR.**

If you take away one thing from this book, let it be the tremendous power of the most basic fundamentals of health: stress management, proper sleep, adequate calorie intake, proper exercise recovery, plenty of time outdoors, proper hydration, and maintenance of proper body temperature. It may be hard to have so much faith in primitive things in a world full of gene expression research, neuropeptides, hormone receptor sites, exotic superfoods, magical drugs, and experimental therapies. But ultimately we would all be healthier, regardless of our hereditary tendencies and predispositions, if we just honored our instincts, and if we truly honored and perfected the basic elements of good physical function and self-care.

We wish you the best
in all your health endeavors!

Dr. Garrett Smith and Matt Stone

You can read more from us and stay tuned to our ongoing research at
www.180degreehealth.com.

REFERENCES

Part One: Stress

Books

Farris, Russell, and Per Marin. *The Potbelly Syndrome*. Laguna Beach, CA: Basic Health Publications, 2006.

Jackson, Grace E. *Rethinking Psychiatric Drugs: A Guide for Informed Consent*. AuthorHouse, 2005.

Keys, Ancel, et al. *The Biology of Human Starvation*. Minneapolis: University of Minnesota Press, 1950.

McCarrison, Robert. *Studies in Deficiency Disease*. London: Henry Frowde and Hodder and Stoughton, 1921.

Rogers, Amber. *Taking Up Space: A Guide to Escaping the Diet Maze*. Ebook. 2013.

Sapolsky, Robert. *Why Zebras Don't Get Ulcers: The Acclaimed Guide to Stress, Stress-Related Diseases, and Coping*. New York: Macmillan, 2004.

Selye, Hans. *The Stress of Life*. New York: McGraw-Hill, 1976.

Talbott, Shawn. *The Cortisol Connection*. Alameda, CA: Hunter House, 2007.

Wiley, T. S. *Lights Out: Sleep, Sugar, and Survival*. New York: Pocket Books, 2000.

Studies

Farshchi, H. R., M. A. Taylor, and I. A. Macdonald. "Beneficial Metabolic Effects of Regular Meal Frequency on Dietary Thermogenesis, Insulin Sensitivity, and Fasting Lipid Profiles in Healthy Obese Women." *American*

Journal of Clinical Nutrition 81 (2005):16–24. http://ajcn.nutrition.org/content/81/1/16.abstract.

Melamed, Samuel, PhD, and Shelly Bruhis. "The Effects of Chronic Industrial Noise Exposure on Urinary Cortisol, Fatigue, and Irritability: A Controlled Field Experiment." *Journal of Occupational & Environmental Medicine* 38, issue 3 (March 1996): 252–256. http://journals.lww.com/joem/Abstract/1996/03000/The_Effects_of_Chronic_Industrial_Noise_Exposure.9.aspx.

Tomiyama, A. Janet, PhD, Traci Mann, PhD, Danielle Vinas, BA, et al. "Low Calorie Dieting Increases Cortisol." *Psychosomatic Medicine* 72, no. 4 (May 2010): 357–364. http://www.ncbi.nlm.nih.gov/pmc/articles/PMC2895000/.

Ward, Alexandra M. V., Caroline H. D. Fall, Claudia E. Stein, et al. "Cortisol and the Metabolic Syndrome in South Asians." *Clinical Endocrinology (Oxford)*. 58, no. 4 (April 2003): 500–505. http://www.ncbi.nlm.nih.gov/pmc/articles/PMC3405820/.

Part Two: **Nutrition**

Books

Barnes, Broda. *Hypothyroidism: The Unsuspecting Illness*. New York: Harper & Row, 1976.

———. *Solved: The Riddle of Heart Attacks*. Fort Collins, CO: Robinson Press, 1976.

———. *Hope for Hypoglycemia*. Fort Collins, CO: Robinson Press, 1978.

Campos, Paul. *The Obesity Myth*. New York: Gotham Books, 2004.

Chilton, Floyd H. *Inflammation Nation*. New York: Fireside, 2007.

Cochran, Gregory, and Henry Harpending. *The 10,000 Year Explosion*. New York: Basic Books, 2009.

Keys, Ancel, et al. *The Biology of Human Starvation*. Minneapolis: University of Minnesota Press, 1950.

Lindeberg, Staffan. *Food and Western Disease*. West Sussex, UK: Wiley-Blackwell, 2010.

McCully, Kilmer S. *The Homocysteine Revolution*. New Canaan, CT: Keats Publishing, 1997.

Pimentel, Mark. *A New IBS Solution*. Sherman Oaks, CA: Health Point Press, 2006.

Starr, Mark. *Hypothyroidism Type II*. Columbia, MO: Mark Starr Trust, 2005.

Tribole, Evelyn, and Elyse Resch. *Intuitive Eating.* New York: St. Martin's Press, 1995.

Wrangham, Richard. *Catching Fire.* New York: Basic Books, 2009.

Studies

Ailhaud, Gérard, Florence Massiera, Pierre Weill, et al. "Temporal Changes in Dietary Fats: Role of n-6 Polyunsaturated Fatty Acids in Excessive Adipose Tissue Development and Relationship to Obesity." *Progress in Lipid Research* 45 (2006): 203–236.

Bixler, David, Joseph Muhler, and William Shafer. "The Relationship between the Histology of the Thyroid and the Salivary Glands and the Incidence of Dental Caries in the Rat." Indiana University School of Dentistry (July 12, 1956). http://jdr.sagepub.com/content/36/4/571.extract.

Dhup, S., R. K. Dadhich, P. E. Porporato, and P. Sonveaux. "Multiple Biological Activities of Lactic Acid in Cancer: Influences on Tumor Growth, Angiogenesis and Metastasis." *Curr Pharm Des* 18, no. 10 (2012): 1319–1330. http://www.ncbi.nlm.nih.gov/pubmed/22360558.

Elliott, Paul. "Sodium Intakes around the World." Background document prepared for the Forum and Technical Meeting on Reducing Salt Intake in Populations. Paris: October 5–7, 2006. http://www.who.int/dietphysicalactivity/Elliot-brown-2007.pdf.

Lopez-Torres, Monica, and Gustavo Barja. "Lowered Methionine Ingestion As Responsible for the Decrease in Rodent Mitochondrial Oxidative Stress in Protein and Dietary Restriction: Possible Implications for Humans." *Biochimica et Biophysica Acta* 1780, no. 11 (2008): 1337–1347. http://cat.inist.fr/?aModele=afficheN&cpsidt=20677212.

Jenkins, D. J., T. M. Wolever, V. Vuksan, et al. "Nibbling versus Gorging: Metabolic Advantages of Increased Meal Frequency." *New England Journal of Medicine* 321, no. 14 (October 1989): 929–934. http://www.ncbi.nlm.nih.gov/pubmed/2674713.

Malik, R., and H. Hodgson. "The Relationship between the Thyroid Gland and the Liver." *Oxford Journals, Medicine, QJM: An International Journal of Medicine* 95, issue 9 (): 559–569. http://qjmed.oxfordjournals.org/content/95/9/559.full.

Matarese, G. "Leptin and the Immune System: How Nutritional Status Influences the Immune Response." *Eur Cytokine Netw* 11, no. 1 (March 2000): 7–14. http://www.ncbi.nlm.nih.gov/pubmed/10705294.

Safer, Joshua D., Tara M. Crawford, and Michael F. Holick. "A Role for Thyroid Hormone in Wound Healing through Keratin Gene Expression." Section of Endocrinology, Department of Medicine, Boston University School of Medicine, Boston, Massachusetts 02118. http://endo.endojournals.org/content/145/5/2357.full.pdf.

Sagara, K., T. Shimada, S. Fujiyama, and T. Sato. "Serum Gastrin Levels in Patients with Thyroid Dysfunction." *Gastrologia Japonica* 18, no. 2 (April 1983): 79–83. http://www.ncbi.nlm.nih.gov/pubmed/6852440.

Seeds, Michael C., Kristina K. Peachman, David L. Bowton, et al. "Regulation of Arachidonate Remodeling Enzymes Impacts Eosinophil Survival during Allergic Asthma." *American Journal of Respiratory Cell Molecular Biology* 41, no. 3 (September 2009): 358–366. http://www.ncbi.nlm.nih.gov/pmc/articles/PMC2742755/.

Sharma, Sunil, and Mani Kavuru. "Sleep and Metabolism: An Overview." Division of Pulmonary, Critical Care and Sleep Medicine, Department of Internal Medicine, Brody School of Medicine, Greenville, 27834 NC (April 28, 2010). http://www.hindawi.com/journals/ije/2010/270832/.

Speakman, John R. "Body Size, Energy Metabolism and Life Span." *Journal of Experimental Biology* (February 2005): 1717-1730. http://jeb.biologists.org/content/208/9/1717.full.

Stolarz-Skrzypek, Katarzyna, et al. "Fatal and Nonfatal Outcomes, Incidence of Hypertension, and Blood Pressure Changes in Relation to Urinary Sodium Excretion." *Journal of the American Medical Association* 305, no. 17 (2011): 1777–1785. doi:10.1001/jama.2011.574. http://jama.jamanetwork.com/article.aspx?articleid=899663.

Todar, Kenneth. "Bacterial Endotoxin," cited in *Todar's Online Textbook of Bacteriology.* http://textbookofbacteriology.net/endotoxin.html.

Online Articles

Sloths: http://www.wildernessclassroom.com/www/schoolhouse/rainforest_library/animal_library/sloth.htm

The Relationship Between Progesterone and Thyroid: http://www.health-truth.com/126.php

Hypothyroid Low Testosterone: http://www.mytestosteronetherapy.com/hypothyroid-low-testosterone/

Natural Testosterone Enhancement: http://180degreehealth.com/2011/03/natural-testosterone-enhancement

Linking Thyroid Problems, Anemia, Fatigue, and Loss of Cognitive Ability: http://www.wellnessresources.com/health/articles/linking_thyroid_problems_anemia_fatigue_and_loss_of_cognitive_ability/

Thyroid, Blood Sugar, and Metabolic Syndrome: http://chriskresser.com/thyroid-blood-sugar-metabolic-syndrome

Carbohydrate Requirements for Exercise http://www.nutrition411.com/ce_pdf/CarbohydrateRequirementsforExercise.pdf

Barbecue Chips Nutrition Data: http://nutritiondata.self.com/facts/snacks/5363/2

Average American Salt Intake: http://www.cdc.gov/features/dssodium/

Thyroid Deficiency and Common Health Problems: http://180degreehealth.com/2013/05/thyroid-deficiency-and-common-health-problems

Movies

The Science of Sex Appeal: (January, 2010). http://www.imdb.com/title/tt1309188/.

Part Three: Exercise

Studies

Boecker, H., et al. "The Runner's High: Opioidergic Mechanisms in the Human Brain." *Cerebral Cortex* 18, no. 11 (November 2008): 2523–2531. http://cercor.oxfordjournals.org/content/18/11/2523.long.

Calogero, A. E., et al. "Environmental Car Exhaust Pollution Damages Human Sperm Chromatin and DNA." *Journal of Endocrinological Investigation* 34, no. 6 (June 2011): e139–143. http://www.ncbi.nlm.nih.gov/pubmed/20959722.

Deinzer, R., et al. "Adrenocortical Responses to Repeated Parachute Jumping and Subsequent h-CRH Challenge in Inexperienced Healthy Subjects." http://www.ncbi.nlm.nih.gov/pubmed/9108568.

Grissom, N., and S. Bhatnagar. "Habituation to Repeated Stress: Get Used to It." *Neurobiology of Learning and Memory* 92, no. 2 (September 2009): 215–224. http://www.ncbi.nlm.nih.gov/pubmed/18667167.

Morton, A. R., et al. "Comparison of Maximal Oxygen Consumption with Oral and Nasal Breathing." *Australian Journal of Science and Medicine in Sport* 27, no. 3 (September 1995): 51–55. http://www.ncbi.nlm.nih.gov/pubmed/8599744.

Scheef, L., et al. "An fMRI Study on the Acute Effects of Exercise on Pain Processing in Trained Athletes." *Pain* 153, no. 8 (August 2012): 1702–1714. http://www.ncbi.nlm.nih.gov/pubmed/22704853.

Takeda, K., et al. "Endocrine-Disrupting Activity of Chemicals in Diesel Exhaust and Diesel Exhaust Particles." *Environmental Science* 11, no. 1 (2004): 33–45. http://www.ncbi.nlm.nih.gov/pubmed/15746887.

Wood, R. J., and A. R. Morton. "Arterial Oxygen Saturation and Peak VO2 during Nasal and Oral Breathing." Proceedings of the American College of Sports Medicine Annual Conference, Medicine and Science in Sport and Exercise. Supplement to Vol 27, no. 5, pS2 (May 1995):. http://www.topendsports.com/resources/research/nasal-oral-breathing.htm.

Online Articles

Longest-lived People and Exercise: http://www.bluezones.com/ and https://en.wikipedia.org/wiki/Jeanne_Calment

Physical Movement and Brain Development: http://www.ted.com/talks/daniel_wolpert_the_real_reason_for_brains.html and

http://www.youtube.com/watch?v=LdDnPYr6R0o

Adrenaline Addiction:

http://www.psychologytoday.com/blog/the-playing-field/200803/the-addicitve-nature-adrenaline-sport

Metabolic Conditioning: http://www.t-nation.com/free_online_article/most_recent/blood_and_chalk_jim_wendler_talks_big_weights_volume_eight and

http://www.t-nation.com/free_online_article/most_recent/conditioning_is_a_sham and

http://70sbig.com/blog/category/content/conditioning/ and

http://anthonymychal.com/wp-content/uploads/2012/05/TheMythofHIIT.pdf

Maffetone Heart Rate Formula: http://philmaffetone.com/180formula.cfm

Vomiting from Exercise: http://www.phase5fitness.com/wp/wp-content/uploads/2012/02/cardio-redux.pdf

Jim Wendler's 5/3/1 Lifting Program: http://www.flexcart.com/members/elitefts/default.asp?m=PD&pid=2976 http://www.flexcart.com/members/elitefts/default.asp?m=PD&pid=2976

Ladders: http://beyondstrong.typepad.com/shafsblog/2007/05/a_primer_on_lad.html

Bulgarian Weight Lifter Training: http://www.t-nation.com/free_online_ article/most_recent/maxing_on_squats_and_deadlifts_every_day

Negative Health Effects of Mouth Breathing: http://www.functionalps.com/ blog/2012/11/30/adverse-effects-of-mouth-breathing/

Breathing and Exercise: http://www.normalbreathing.com/c-effects-of-exercise-on-the-respiratory-system.php

Part Four: Sleep and Recovery

Studies

Grounding/Earthing

Brown, D., et al. "Pilot Study on the Effect of Grounding on Delayed-Onset Muscle Soreness." *Journal of Alternative and Complementary Medicine* 16, no. 3 (March 2010): 265–273. http://www.ncbi.nlm.nih.gov/pubmed/20192911.

Chevalier, G. "Changes in Pulse Rate, Respiratory Rate, Blood Oxygenation, Perfusion Index, Skin Conductance, and Their Variability Induced during and after Grounding Human Subjects for 40 Minutes." *Journal of Alternative and Complementary Medicine* 16, no. 1 (January 2010): 81–87. http://www. earthinginstitute.net/studies/earthing_pulse_rate.pdf.

Chevalier, G., et al. "Earthing: Health Implications of Reconnecting the Human Body to the Earth's Surface Electrons." *Journal of Environmental Public Health* (2012): 291541. http://www.ncbi.nlm.nih.gov/pmc/articles/ PMC3265077/.

———. "Earthing (Grounding) the Human Body Reduces Blood Viscosity—A Major Factor in Cardiovascular Disease." *Journal of Alternative and Complementary Medicine* 19, no. 2 (February 2013): 102–110. http:// online.liebertpub.com/doi/pdf/10.1089/acm.2011.0820.

Chevalier, G., and S. Sinatra. "Emotional Stress, Heart Rate Variability, Grounding, and Improved Autonomic Tone: Clinical Applications." *Integrative Medicine* 10, no. 3 (June/July 2011): 16-21. http://imjournal.com/ pdfarticles/IMCJ10_3_p16_24chevalier.pdf.

Ghaly, M., and D. Teplitz. "The Biologic Effects of Grounding the Human Body during Sleep As Measured by Cortisol Levels and Subjective Reporting of Sleep, Pain, and Stress." *Journal of Alternative and Complementary Medicine* 10, no. 5 (October 2004): 767–776. http://www.ncbi.nlm.nih.gov/ pubmed/15650465.

Oschman, J. L. "Can Electrons Act As Antioxidants? A Review and Commentary." *Journal of Alternative and Complementary Medicine* 13, no. 9 (November 2007): 955–967. http://www.ncbi.nlm.nih.gov/pubmed/18047442.

Sokal, K., and P. Sokal. "Earthing the Human Body Influences Physiologic Processes." *Journal of Alternative and Complementary Medicine* 17, no. 4 (April 2011): 301–308. http://www.ncbi.nlm.nih.gov/pmc/articles/ PMC3154031/.

———. "The Neuromodulative Role of Earthing." *Medical Hypotheses* 77, no. 5 (November 2011): 824–826. http://www.ncbi.nlm.nih.gov/ pubmed/21856083.

———. "Earthing the Human Organism Influences Bioelectrical Processes." *Journal of Alternative and Complementary Medicine* 18, no. 3 (March 2012): 229–234. http://www.ncbi.nlm.nih.gov/pubmed/22420736.

Forest Bathing

Kamioka, H., et al. "A Systematic Review of Randomized Controlled Trials on Curative and Health Enhancement Effects of Forest Therapy." *Psychology Research and Behavior Management* 5 (2012): 85–95. http://www.ncbi.nlm. nih.gov/pmc/articles/PMC3414249/.

Karjalainen, E., et al. "Promoting Human Health through Forests: Overview and Major Challenges." *Environmental Health and Preventive Medicine* 15, no. 1 (January 2010): 1–8.

http://www.ncbi.nlm.nih.gov/pmc/articles/PMC2793342/.

Lee, J., et al. "Effect of Forest Bathing on Physiological and Psychological Responses in Young Japanese Male Subjects." *Public Health* 125, no. 2 (February 2011): 93–100. http://www.ncbi.nlm.nih.gov/pubmed/21288543.

Li, Q., et al. "Forest Bathing Enhances Human Natural Killer Activity and Expression of Anti-Cancer Proteins." *International Journal of Immunopathology and Pharmacology* 20, no. 2, Supplement 2 (April–June 2007): 3–8. http://www.ncbi.nlm.nih.gov/pubmed/17903349.

———. "A Forest Bathing Trip Increases Human Natural Killer Activity and Expression of Anti-Cancer Proteins in Female Subjects." *Journal of Biological Regulators and Homeostatic Agents* 22, no. 1 (January–March 2008): 45–55. http://www.ncbi.nlm.nih.gov/pubmed/18394317.

———. "Visiting a Forest, But Not a City, Increases Human Natural Killer Activity and Expression of Anti-Cancer Proteins." *International Journal of*

Immunopathology and Pharmacology 21, no. 1 (January–March 2008): 117–127. http://www.ncbi.nlm.nih.gov/pubmed/18336737.

———. "Effect of Forest Bathing Trips on Human Immune Function." *Environmental Health and Preventive Medicine* 15, no. 1 (January 2010): 9–17. http://www.ncbi.nlm.nih.gov/pmc/articles/PMC2793341/.

Mao, G. X., et al. "Effects of Short-Term Forest Bathing on Human Health in a Broad-Leaved Evergreen Forest in Zhejiang Province, China." *Biomedical Environmental Science* 25, no. 3 (June 2012): 317–324. http://www.besjournal.com/Articles/Archive/archive/No3/201207/t20120712_64252.html.

———. "Therapeutic Effect of Forest Bathing on Human Hypertension in the Elderly." *Journal of Cardiology* 60, no. 6 (December 2012): 495–502. http://www.ncbi.nlm.nih.gov/pubmed/22948092.

Morita, E., et al. "Psychological Effects of Forest Environments on Healthy Adults: *Shinrin-yoku* (Forest-Air Bathing, Walking) As a Possible Method of Stress Reduction." *Public Health* 121, no. 1 (January 2007): 54–63. http://www.ncbi.nlm.nih.gov/pubmed/17055544.

Ohira, H., et al. "Effect of *Shinrin-yoku* (Forest-Air Bathing and Walking) on Mental and Physical Health." *Bulletin of Tokai Women's College* 19 (1999): 217–232.

Ohtsuka, Y., et al. "*Shinrin-yoku* (Forest-Air Bathing and Walking) Effectively Decreases Blood Glucose Levels in Diabetic Patients." *International Journal of Biometeorology* 41, no. 3 (February 1998): 125–127. http://www.ncbi.nlm.nih.gov/pubmed/9531856.

Park, B. J., et al. "The Physiological Effects of *Shinrin-yoku* (Taking in the Forest Atmosphere or Forest Bathing): Evidence from Field Experiments in 24 Forests across Japan." *Environmental Health and Preventive Medicine* 15, no. 1 (January 2010): 18–26. http://www.ncbi.nlm.nih.gov/pmc/articles/PMC2793346/.

Thompson, Coon J., et al. "Does Participating in Physical Activity in Outdoor Natural Environments Have a Greater Effect on Physical and Mental Wellbeing Than Physical Activity Indoors? A Systematic Review." *Environmental Science and Technology* 45, no. 5 (March 2011): 1761–1772. http://www.ncbi.nlm.nih.gov/pubmed/21291246.

Tsunetsugu, Y., et al. "Trends in Research Related to 'Shinrin-yoku' (Taking in the Forest Atmosphere or Forest Bathing) in Japan." *Environmental Health and Preventive Medicine* 15, no. 1 (January 2010): 27–37. http://www.ncbi.nlm.nih.gov/pmc/articles/PMC2793347/#CR40.

Yamaguchi, M., et al. "The Effects of Exercise in Forest and Urban Environments on Sympathetic Nervous Activity of Normal Young Adults." *Journal of International Medical Research* 34, no. 2 (March–April 2006): 152–159. http://www.ncbi.nlm.nih.gov/pubmed/16749410.

EMFs and RFR

FDA on Cellular: http://www.fda.gov/Radiation-EmittingProducts/RadiationEmittingProductsandProcedures/HomeBusinessandEntertainment/CellPhones/ucm116282.htm

FCC on Cellular: http://www.fcc.gov/guides/wireless-devices-and-health-concerns

World Health Organization on Tobacco Industry Cover-up: http://www.who.int/tobacco/media/en/TobaccoExplained.pdf

The BioInitiative Report: http://www.bioinitiative.org

BioInitiative Report's RFR Research Chart: http://www.bioinitiative.org/rf-color-charts/

Environmental Working Group's Executive Summary on RFR: http://www.ewg.org/cellphoneradiation/executivesummary/

Suppressed Environmental Protection Agency RFR Guidelines: http://electromagnetichealth.org/media-stories/#Exposure-Guidelines

INDEX